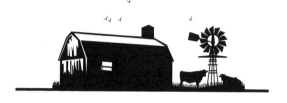

WHERE THE GRASS GROWS GREENER

Inspirational Stories from
Lancaster County Veterinarian

BOB STOLTZFUS

Where the Grass Grows Greener
by Bob Stoltzfus

Copyright © 2024
All rights reserved.

Library of Congress Control Number: 2024932112
International Standard Book Number: 978-1-60126-909-6

Masthof Press
219 Mill Road | Morgantown, PA 19543-9516
www.Masthof.com

I dedicate this book to my wife, Joyce,
and to my daughters, Abigail and Juliann, to my son Kendal,
and to their families and descendants. They have been with
me through the good and bad times.
God bless you all.

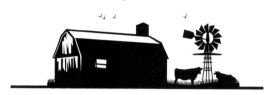

TABLE OF CONTENTS

What Is This Book?

My childhood years were spent growing up on a dairy farm in Pennsylvania. My father was a hardworking parent that rose early in the day to milk cows, work the farm, and then milk the cows again finishing late in the day. This was his routine 7 days a week all year long. The growing season was particularly busy as he worked the day tilling the soil, planting the crops, then harvesting and storing them for feeding the cows during the winter. The off season was less busy allowing him some time during the day to plan, manage the business, and maintain and repair equipment.

As a child I, too, helped as I was able to for my age. Some of my earliest memories consist of steering a Farmal H tractor slowly in a field while he and my older brothers picked up bales of hay. I was too small to reach the clutch and brake pedals. My father would put the tractor in first gear, throttle down the engine so that the tractor and wagon would just creep along. Then he would sit me up on the seat, step off the tractor, and tell me to steer the tractor so that he and my older brothers could load the wagon with bales of hay as he guided me through the long rows of hay bales lying on the ground. I felt important.

As I grew older, my responsibilities increased. I became more involved in helping with all the chores. I loved field work. I can remember driving tractor late at night under the dark sky with the whole universe of stars, constellations, and the roar of the tractor engine pulling an implement through the fields. To this day, I am reminded of those times when I see the constellations of Orion and the Big and Little Dippers in the night sky.

During my early school years, I took an interest in feeding the young calves in the barn. I would get up early before school to feed the calves. I would run back to the house to eat a bowl of cheerios, get dressed for school, and catch the school bus for the ride to school. I learned to milk the cows and tend to their needs. I had favorite cows. Some were part of the family. Some were mean and one had to be careful around them. They had personalities and when you spend a lot of time with cows, you get to know them as individuals. They all had names. They all had appointed stalls in the barn.

I loved the farm and as any young boy would, I dreamed of following in my father's footsteps as a dairy farmer. I am not sure when it started but at some point in my life I developed a dream of spending my adult life as a large animal veterinarian. I never expected to achieve that dream.

As I look back on my years of education, I remember hating school. The best day of school was the last day before summer vacation. Yet I always did well in my studies. I had a good memory and attention to detail that carried me along with minimal effort. That was true all through elementary and high school. The farm taught me a strong work ethic. Never give up and stay on task until the job is finished.

My father encouraged me to attend college so I enrolled in a four-year liberal arts college. I spent the first year of college having fun while still managing to maintain passing grades without my full effort.

The second year required me to be more studious and I learned to love the science courses. I studied hard and did very well in them. I also met the love of my life and future wife, Joyce. True to her name, she brought joy to my life. She was an excellent student and studied a lot. We studied together. It gave me an excuse to be with her. If I had to study to be with her, so be it. My grades got better and I learned how to be more studious and take life and the future more seriously. I loved science and took as many of those courses as I could. The dream of attending veterinary school became more of a possibility.

My third year of college is where it got serious. I took an organic chemistry course taught by a professor who demanded your best performance. He seemed to enjoy the task of challenging students to achieve their fullest potential. It forced me to learn how to study and prepare well for tests. I credit that professor for teaching me to be a student and give it my best effort. Never give up. I did very well in his course, assisted by the time studying with Joyce.

My fourth year of college continued the science curriculum, which I loved. I did very well. Now it was time to plan. The dream of veterinary school became more realistic. I sent my application. There were 35 applicants for every position at the University of Pennsylvania School of Veterinary Medicine.

After graduation from college, Joyce and I were married and we started our lives together. We moved into an apartment. I worked with my father on the dairy farm and Joyce worked in a local hospital. The future was uncertain. The two of us newlyweds just enjoyed our time together without much concern for where life would take us. It seemed like our lives would continue on the dairy farm.

Months later, I got my rejection letter from the Veterinary School. It confirmed our destiny on the dairy farm. I showed the letter to my father. He pushed me not to become discouraged. He encouraged me to persist with the pursuit of my dreams. Do not give up. He pushed me to make an appointment with the Dean of Admissions to discover what I needed to do to advance my application. Joyce was also supportive of pushing forward.

My father and I drove to Philadelphia and I sat with the Dean of Admissions. He explained to me how difficult it was for admission to the Veterinary School. Most applicants are not accepted until their third application. Meanwhile I should continue to take science courses at a college and keep applying.

I took his advice and registered for a full load of science courses at a local reputable college while working with my father on the dairy farm. I would get up early in the morning to help milk the cows. Then it was off to college for the day. In the evening, I would return home to milk the cows again and complete my studies. My grades were excellent because I loved the science courses. I applied again to the Veterinary School. After completing a year of a full science curriculum, I was admitted to the Veterinary School on my third application.

Veterinary school was tough going. It required an all-out effort to keep up with the studies. Joyce found work as a bookkeeper to support us. She was awesome. She, too, had grown up on a dairy farm and had a strong work ethic. I never would have made it through those difficult times without her. Finances were lean and I borrowed funds to pay the school bills.

To complicate matters, my father was killed in a farm accident the week before my first set of final exams. He had already sold the milking cows that previous summer before I went off to school. Now I was tasked with attending veterinary school and studying during the week and tending to what had to be done to maintain the farm on weekends. Most of the farm work consisted of crop work done in the summers when school was out of session. I did this and nothing else for the first three years of veterinary school. These were difficult times for Joyce as well. We did not spend much quality time together. It was complicated by the loss of my father and my mother's dependence on me to run the farm. Joyce stuck with me through it all.

I always appreciated the fact that my father unselfishly placed my dream of being a veterinarian ahead of his dream of passing the farm off to me and the two of us working together on the farm. It may have cost him his life. I am sobered by that act of unselfishness. It is parental love.

I have been a large animal veterinarian for most of my life. It has been very good to me. I prefer the outdoors. Do not put me in an office cubicle. I offer my services to both large corporate farms and small Amish farms in south central Pennsylvania. I love working with farm people and becoming an important part of their business. The most gratifying and encouraging thing for me is to make my clients better and more successful at what they do. Money cannot buy that kind of satisfaction. It comes from interacting with people. They become more than just clients. They are friends. We get to see and know each other as we really are. We share experiences together, some quite humorous and some more serious.

Over the years, I have accumulated a memory database of many such experiences. I find people love to hear stories of these farm experiences. The ones they love the most are the self-deprecating stories. People love to hear the details of how I made a fool out of myself (grin).

So what is this book? This book is a compilation of many of those memories intertwined with a life lesson. It is a collection of experiences I want to remember. Most chapters begin with a story that illustrates some aspect of life. Following the story is a discourse of my thoughts illustrated by the story. These may stimulate the reader to examine their own thoughts and beliefs. Some may agree, some will disagree. I hope that all will think about their own lives and beliefs in some fashion. I am not a philosopher or a theologian. I am just me, a task and detail-oriented, pragmatist. This book is a combination of my memoirs as a veterinarian and a challenge to the reader to think about what is important in their own lives.

I remember an incident that happened with our neighboring farmers when I was very young. They had moved to the country from New York City to take up the rural lifestyle. They raised sheep. Occasionally a group of their sheep would crawl through the border fence between our farms and graze in our pasture. My mother would call them on our party line phone and inform them that their sheep had escaped. She did not want the sheep to wander off and become lost. The neighbors would apologize and retrieve their sheep.

On one occasion my mother joked that, she guessed the grass was greener on the other side of their fence. This comes from an old Pennsylvania Dutch expression that "The grass is always greener on the other side of the fence." It seems that livestock will often reach as far as they can through a woven wire fence to reach that special blade of grass just beyond their reach. It illustrates that subliminal urge we all have to acquire something not readily available. There is plenty of grass on our side of the fence. Nevertheless, we want that which at first seems beyond our ability to reach.

To continue the story, our neighbors were offended at the suggestion that our grass was better than their grass. Apparently, they were not familiar with that old expression. It took an explanation to familiarize them with that aspect of country life.

As one reads this book, I hope that they are engaged to long for what is not readily apparent, to search beyond their self-imposed barriers, and challenged to look beyond the obvious to acquire a life beyond their expectations, where the grass grows greener. I hope the reader will use it as a springboard to examine their own beliefs and priorities about what is important in life. Do not be constrained by the barriers you face. The greatest obstacle to spiritual development is the failure to recognize the existence of the spiritual reality. The grass really is greener on the other side of the fence.

CHAPTER 1

Just Another Day

Misty summer evenings are great for loafing around the house or just grabbing a good book and sinking into your favorite chair. Today is Saturday and it is raining. It is not a drenching rain but rather a drifting mist that makes everything soaking wet. Farmers call this "perfect corn grow'n weath'r." Some say that one can actually hear the corn creak as the stalks grow. The sight of a large field of dark green and shiny corn leaves soaking up the energy from the sun is always a pleasant reminder of the importance of agriculture in our lives. Often taken for granted, we depend upon our farmers for the food on our tables every day. Because modern agriculture is so efficient in the production of our food, it has set most of our population free from the daily toils of tilling the earth and tending the animals. Instead, we pursue other interests in making our lives more fun filled, productive, and automated.

In the midst of the evening solitude, my ringing phone breaks the peace of this Saturday evening. The message is that Paul has a "cow down." I have come to accept these intrusions as a necessary part of the job. Providing emergency service means you make yourself available to help as the need arises at any time of day or night. Dairy cows never take a break. Dairy producers milk cows every day on a regular 24-hour schedule. Most of the smaller family herds milk twice a day with 12 hours between the milkings. The schedules often are something like 4 a.m. and 4 p.m. The larger herds run their milking parlors almost around the clock with just enough time between milkings to clean and sanitize the parlor and equipment before the start of the next milking.

When people are working with their cows, they see the health problems that need immediate attention and so they call the Vet. Emergency calls come at any time, but they usually occur in the early morning or evening when workers are near the cows.

The most common cause for a "cow down" is "milk fever." Its name does not describe its cause. Cows with milk fever are unable to stand because they lose voluntary muscle control due to a low serum calcium level. They also lose control of their ability to regulate their body temperature. If they are out in the sun on a hot summer day, their body temperature will rise and they will have a fever. If they are in the shade on a cold winter morning their body temperature will be below normal. Fever is not necessarily a part of the disease. Milk fever occurs within hours of a cow giving birth to a calf. With the demand for the production of milk after calving, some cows are unable to keep their level of calcium in the blood above a level necessary for vital functions. Consequently, their blood calcium drops, they lose control of their muscles, become shaky, lay down, and are unable to rise to their feet again. As the disease continues, the cow will lie over on her side and accumulate gas in her stomach. The syndrome progresses over several hours until it ends with death.

When Paul called for a "cow down," I suspected it was probably a cow with milk fever. Treating these cows by giving them a dose of calcium gluconate in their jugular vein is easy and usually yields a rewarding result within minutes of the treatment. These cows literally respond to the treatment while the liquid is flowing into their jugular vein. The response is spectacular. A cow can be down on her side with her stomach full of air, struggling to breath, and near to death. While receiving the treatment she will begin to "burp" off the gas. Within minutes of receiving the full dose, she may rise to her feet and walk away as though nothing ever happened.

I change into my work clothes, put on a pair of clean coveralls, get into my vehicle, and begin the drive out to Paul's farm. The mist is heavy as it drifts down from the sky and soaks every surface with water. I put the windshield wipers on delay as I make my way out my driveway to the main road. Traffic is light. Most people do not venture out on this dreary evening. It is getting late in the evening as the sun is about to sink below the western horizon. It is about a fifteen-minute drive to his farm.

As I turn into Paul's farm lane, I can see that the lights are still on in the barn. Apparently, he is just finishing up with the evening chores. The first thing I do when arriving on a farm is go to the milk house and fill a stainless steel bucket with clean, warm water.

I enjoy Paul. I am not one that demands to be addressed by my proper title. As a large animal veterinarian, I know my clients on a first-name basis. Most address me as "Dr. Bob." Paul is different. He is always very respectful with a serious demeanor. He always addresses me as "Doctor." He is a man of short stature in the sixth decade of life. His face shows the ravages and wrinkles of many hard days of work in the sun. His wrinkles have wrinkles. His voice is rough and crackly. As I walk into the barn carrying my clean bucket of water, I see Paul kneeling beside a cow to remove the milking machine. I start the conversation with a simple "Hi Paul."

He slowly rises from his position and takes a few short and stiff steps to greet me.

"Good evening Doctor," he responds as a gentile grin creeps across his tired face.

"Where is the cow that is down?" I ask.

"Well Doctor, I'm very sorry but she is not in the barn. She is out in the back pasture."

"When did she calve?"

"Must have been some time during this afternoon. I went out to the pasture this evening and found her down with a calf by her side."

"Okay, I suspect that she may have milk fever. I'll just drive my car out to her in the back pasture."

"Oh no Doctor. That will not be possible. The pasture is very hilly and rocky. You will not be able to drive your car to her. I'll take you there myself."

He is very polite but insists that he has a better plan. I quietly and respectfully agree to travel to the down cow in his pasture by his mode of transportation. I make a quick trip back to my car to retrieve the materials and medicines that I will need to treat the cow.

"Come on out behind the barn," Paul instructed.

As I round the barn, I see that he has completed preparations for my arrival. True to his polite nature, he has prepared the best of accommodations for me. He hooked his largest farm tractor to a tiny garden trailer. It is a small garden trailer that homeowners use to haul leaves around their yard. Inside the trailer is an old rusty lawn chair. It is an aluminum-folding chair with green and yellow plastic web. The web is frayed after many years of use.

"Here Doctor, have a seat in the trailer. I'll take you out to treat the cow."

As I step into the trailer, he hands me an umbrella.

"Here, hold this above your head so that you don't get wet."

It is an umbrella that bears the scars of many years of use. It has large obnoxious daisy-like red flowers in a print pattern. I desperately want to resist. I am not a fragile daisy that needs pampering. I am accustomed to getting wet, slimy, and dirty. I can take the abuse. I rather enjoy it. It has got to be much healthier than a proper sport coat, white shirt and tie. However, Paul insists. He is so apologetic for calling me to his farm on a misty summer evening that I cannot resist. I take a seat on the old rusty and frayed lawn chair. I open the gaudy umbrella and proudly hoist it high above my head. I might as well go in style. Thank God, no one is watching.

Paul proudly climbed up into his big tractor equipped with all the latest creature comforts, started the mighty engine, slid it into gear and we were off to the back pasture. He is pleased with himself for thinking of all the details necessary to complete this mission.

Instead of driving us out to the pasture behind the barn where no one can see us, he drives the tractor out the driveway and onto the main road. I did not know that he had a pasture in another location. As we proceed down the road, we soon find ourselves on the main street of a small town with houses lining the street. I am not expecting this scenario. It has the appearance of a ceremonial float carrying the queen in a homecoming parade. He is parading me down Main Street, the main attraction, sitting on this ridiculous rusty chair, holding a gaudy umbrella, in a tiny trailer behind a mighty tractor. I drop the umbrella lower until I can scarcely see out from under it, hoping that at least the local folks do not recognize me. I am the new Vet in this farming community. This will make for great fun at the local sandwich shop.

As the tractor picks up speed, the gigantic rear tires began to pick up water from the road and throw it in my direction. The droplets of dirty road filth water are flying high in the air and come drifting down on me from all directions. The umbrella only serves as a canopy to hide me from amused eyes. The tractor has too much power for the load it is pulling. The trailer jumps off the road at the slightest little bump. Any large pothole will be a disaster. With every bump, my chair slides around on the floor of the trailer. I hope that the frayed chair webbing does not rip away from the chair frame and dump the homecoming queen. I plant my feet to brace myself and become one with the bouncing chair while also maintaining a position somewhat near the center of gravity for the trailer. As I focus on maintaining my health, I become oblivious to everything else. I hope my obituary will not be in tomorrow's newspaper.

We slow down. The bouncing stops. The road filth shower fades. We make a right turn off the road. Thank God, this part of the ride is ended. As we are midway through our turn, I look ahead and I am near panic at what I see. It is a cattle guard.

As the domestication of cattle has progressed over the ages, so has the ingenuity of those that care for them. We have gone from shepherds, to stone hedges, to split rail fences, to woven wire, barbed wire, and electric fences. With the use of fences, gates became necessary as a means to enter and exit the fenced area. Therefore, gates have undergone the same metamorphosis as the fences have. As transportation progressed from horses to vehicles, new ideas adapt to the construction of gateways. A cattle guard is a slatted grate of concrete or steel on the surface of the ground that wheels can easily roll across. Cattle hooves cannot walk across the grate. The alternating slats and spaces do not permit proper footing. The benefit is that the operator of a vehicle does not need to stop, disembark from the vehicle to open a gate, and then disembark again to close the gate. Crossing a cattle guard is like driving across a dozen old, rickety, pot holed railroad crossings simultaneously. There is no way to do it without being tossed and bounced in many directions.

I brace myself for the worst, hoping that Paul will not accelerate before hitting the cattle guard. He slows down as we cross it. True to his very respectful nature, he is considerate of my dilemma. The water in my bucket is splashing violently but there is still some water remaining as we successfully reach the far side of the cattle guard.

We enter the realm of traversing the uneven terrain of the pasture in search of the down cow. As we cross over ditches, rocks, and sloping hillsides, my chair and I slide around on the floor of the trailer and bounce off the sides like the ball in a pinball machine.

We finally stop at the bottom of a hill beside a small ditch. I rise to my shaky feet and regain my composure, I notice the cow lying on her side a short distance from us. She is a large black and white cow. She appears to be up in years like her owner. It is my turn to take control of the situation.

The cow is in need of immediate treatment. She is unable to rise. She is lying over on her side and her stomach is full of gas. She looks like a balloon with legs. She is bloated to the degree that breathing has become difficult for her. I grab my intravenous tube and connect it to a 500 ml bottle of calcium gluconate. I place a rope halter on the cow's head and stretch out her neck to expose her jugular vein. I place an intravenous needle in her jugular vein, prime the calcium solution in the IV tube and connect it to the needle already placed in her jugular vein.

As the calcium solution runs slowly into her vein I place my stethoscope over her chest and listen to her heartbeat. Some cows will develop an irregular heartbeat leading to no heartbeat and death while receiving calcium. Therefore, I listen to the heartbeat while giving them calcium. It makes me feel better to hear a regular heartbeat without an arrhythmia. As the medicine slowly drips into her bloodstream, she begins to respond favorably. Her heartbeat is slow and regular. She begins to shake and shiver as she regains the use of her voluntary muscles.

Most cows will take the calcium without any problem. That is the case with this cow. As the solution runs into her vein, I hear her begin to burp the gas from her bloated rumen. By the time I am finished she has belched off most of the gas. I remove the needle from her vein. Paul and I roll the cow up on her sternum so that she is resting comfortably. She belches a few more times. I complete a more thorough exam of her checking for other problems that often accompany this condition. After a few more minutes, she looks much better. With a little encouragement, she rises to her feet. She looks for her calf and begins to take care of it. Treating these cows is usually quite rewarding since they respond so quickly in a brief amount of time. I enjoy the visual image of a mother cow carefully and tenderly caring for her wet, newborn calf.

"Paul. It looks like we got to her in time," I say while collecting my gear.

"Thank you very much Doctor," he says. "I'll give you a ride back to the barn."

The trip back is very much like my maiden voyage. We arrive safe and sound at the barn and exchange pleasantries once again. I wash up and pack my gear. As I slowly wander my vehicle out the driveway, Paul gives me a final farewell wave. I smile, return his wave, and I am on my way.

Thankfully, this farm call has a good outcome. This is my life. It is just another day. As I go about my daily activities, I become rather methodical about each day. Challenges come and go and my responses are preprogrammed based upon my education and experiences. The daily routine consists of being aware of what my senses are detecting. Then I make serial decisions based upon established knowledge and experience to act appropriately to whatever challenge lies before me.

For Paul, myself, and the rest of humanity, our existence consists of receiving information through our five physical senses of sight, taste, hearing, smell, and touch. We then process that information in our brain and formulate an appropriate reaction for our muscles to execute.

We see and hear danger racing toward us. Our brain says danger is imminent, run. Our muscles take action as we flee.

We see and hear someone speaking to us. Our brain processes the thought. We respond by using our voice muscles to speak in return.

This pattern repeats itself all day, every day, as life continues. In a strictly physical manner, we are not a lot different than other animals responding constantly to their sensory input and the needs presented to them by the environment they occupy.

This is the entirety of life for each of us, OR IS IT? Like an iceberg there may be a lot more that we cannot see that lies below the visible surface. Is there more to our existence than just the daily grind to gut out a livelihood of the pursuit of personal wealth and pleasure?

CHAPTER 2

Beyond the Barriers

It is a mild springtime Sunday afternoon. I am sitting in the gate area of Dulles International Airport. I am looking for a middle-aged man wearing a baseball cap. That is my cue to meet up with a gentleman to embark on a service project through USAID and the Farmer-to-Farmer program. His name is John. We are to travel to remote regions of Kazakhstan to provide assistance to their dairy farms.

I have arrived in the gate area early to not miss my contact. There are many middle-aged men wearing baseball caps. Which one is he? I do not know. It is still early so rather than start asking all the middle-aged men wearing baseball caps if their name is John, I just take a seat and wait. There is a high probability that more than one of these men is named John. After a while, a man wearing a baseball cap who looks like he just left his dairy barn walks over to me and introduces himself as John. This is my contact.

John is a dairy farmer from central Pennsylvania. He has a passion to bolster and support several dairies in Kazakhstan. John has made many trips to the country for this purpose. He has several contacts within the country. His passion is Ayrshire cattle. He has brought improved genetics in the form of frozen semen and embryos along with him on these trips. He often brings other industry support personnel with him to add their expertise to the experience.

My role on this trip is to provide nutritional and veterinary support to his project. For a rookie like me he is a welcome mentor to help me adjust to the rigors of the trip and guide me along the way. He gives me many survival tips. An important tip is to always carry a small pack of tissues as emergency bathroom paper since there is no guarantee of it being available where we are going to find ourselves. That turned out to be a valuable tip.

An item in my checked luggage is a large cardboard box containing an ultrasound machine. I will deliver this to a farm that bought it for the reproductive management of their cows.

I face this adventure with intrigue at the opportunity to serve dairy farms outside of my local community and country. Kazakhstan is a former part of the Soviet Union. Kazakhstan is where the Soviets have built some of their nuclear weapons and nuclear weapon launch facilities. In earlier years there were nuclear weapons aimed at the United States from their launch facilities in Kazakhstan, a rather sobering thought. Now I am traveling to the country that had nuclear weapons aimed at my country.

John and I board the first leg of our flight itinerary that eventually will take us to Almaty, the capitol of Kazakhstan. We fly to England and after a short layover travel the final leg of our trip. We arrive in Kazakhstan early in the morning two and a half days later.

As I pass through customs in Almaty, I am aware of the military presence in the area. There are soviet style soldiers with their large military hats watching your every move. I am a bit concerned about getting the large box containing the ultrasound machine through customs.

To add to my concern is the fact that I included in the box a flat of hormones used to synchronize reproductive cycles in dairy cattle. These are gonadotropin releasing hormone (GNRH) and Prostaglandin (PG). They are not part of the ultrasound machine but I was asked to bring them along for the dairies in Kazakhstan. I included them in the ultrasound box hoping that they would look like part of the machine as it passed through the X-ray machine in customs. If the box is opened, the vials will be discovered and I will have some explaining to do. My trip through customs was uneventful as the box remained closed.

The time difference is eleven hours from my home in Pennsylvania. Jet lag sets in compounded by the long trip. We make accommodations for one day at a hotel and then begin our work with the local contacts.

I check into the Hotel Almaty. The hotel room has the necessities, a bed and a small bathroom. There is no heat in the hotel since the city has turned off the steam that it pipes throughout the city to supply heat to the residents and businesses. It is mid-April and like clockwork, this is when they turn off the steam.

Upon arrival at the hotel, I try to take a nap, but my internal time clock is out of sync with the sun and sleep is impossible. Two hours pass and then we gather our crew together for an introductory meeting. John and I have an interpreter, a driver, and Hisa. Hisa is a man that John is working with to build a company that will support dairy farms in his country of Kazakhstan. Hisa is a very kind, gentle, sincere, and generous person. As time passes, I grow to like him very much.

My assigned duties are three-fold. First, I am to look at the nutritional status of their cows and make feeding recommendations for improving health and productivity. Second, I am to converse with the staff on the farms, chat, and compare management and treatments for common health and productivity problems of dairy cows. Third, I am to deliver an ultrasound machine that I brought along on the trip and show them how to use it for the reproductive evaluations of their cattle.

We decide to get started. We travel to a local dairy outside Almaty and meet the farm director, Ivan. Ivan is a middle-aged man, confident in appearance, and happy to show us his farm. He is dressed in a tan-colored three-piece business suit, white button-down collar shirt, and red tie. He first leads us to a pen of heifers that are the subject of his pride. These heifers are soon due to deliver calves from embryos that were transferred into them. On a previous visit, John had brought the embryos along with a veterinarian who specialized in embryo transfer.

That veterinarian recognized the need for proper nutrition, which led to my visit today. Ivan sees the need to improve the genetic production potential of his herd and is insistent about learning as much as he can to improve his dairy herd. Through an interpreter, I dialogue with him answering his many questions as best I can about improving his dairy. I am impressed with his desire to learn and adapt new technologies.

Ivan's farm is a former Russian commune style farm. The barns are constructed of concrete. The cows are tethered in stalls in long rows inside the barn. There is a caretaker for each row of cows. Ventilation in the barns is not ideal but the cows are healthy and in good body condition. These are not Holstein cows like we have in the U.S. They are a dual-purpose dairy and beef cow typical of Russian farms.

We spend a little time learning about his farm. My first impression is that there are no local businesses to support this farm. There are no agricultural supply stores, no feed stores, no grain mills, and no equipment repair shops. The farm is an isolated entity that needs to supply nearly everything from within or travel long distances to acquire needed items and services.

We travel back to the hotel for the evening. Car travel in Kazakhstan is hazardous. The roads are wide but there are no painted lane markings and no speed limits. Traffic accidents are common. It is a free for all with each car competing for favored positions on the roadway. At the red traffic light in Almaty, cars pull up beside each other. When the light turns green, we are in the midst of a drag race as everybody puts the pedal to the metal and the fastest car wins the front position on the highway. That is until someone tries to pass the lead car. Then it is another pedal to the metal drag race.

We make it safely back to the hotel. I go to bed early and manage to fall asleep for a good rest. The next day will soon arrive.

I am aware that the hotel staff watches my every move. I keep my valuables locked away in a suitcase since the staff has access to my room when I am not present. I can tell that they enter the room when I am gone and look through whatever they can access. I feel violated as my personal belongings are none of their business. I make sure there is nothing for them to see by locking everything away from their prying eyes.

We arise early the next morning. Today we board a train to travel to several farms in the far northeast of Kazakhstan near the Russian border of Siberia. After a nice breakfast, buffet style in the hotel, we head to the train station.

Our accommodations on the train consist of a small cabin with two cots and a small window with a venetian blind covering it. I open the blind so that I can see outside. If I have any phobia, it might be claustrophobia. I need space. I like the outdoors. I share the room with John.

The train's travel is constantly interrupted by stops at other train stations along the way. There is a toilet at the rear end of each passenger car. I notice that the train attendants lock the toilet at every station. On my first visit, I discover why they lock them. As I peer down into the toilet opening, I see the railroad ties pass by as we travel. There is no bottom in the toilet. Everything falls through to the tracks below. I would hate to be a track worker on this line. This is the reason they lock the toilets in the train stations.

Mile after mile we travel. Once we are out of the capitol city, there is little activity to look at. As I peer out the window, all I see is mile after mile of gentle rolling unoccupied grassland. There are no buildings, no people, no animals, just grass.

On one occasion, I see a cowboy on horseback tending to a few beef cattle grazing on the grass.

Much of the journey we spend with our hosts in the neighboring cabin conversing on a variety of subjects. I spend many hours talking with Hisa. Hisa speaks English very well so it is nice to visit with someone that does not need an interpreter. He is so eager to learn and be a resource to those he has chosen to serve. Our conversation is not limited to dairy industry issues. We talk about our lives, our hobbies, and our families. We talk about our countries. I find that there is much interest in talking about life in the United States. I am careful not to get into political discussions but rather just talk and learn about our lifestyles.

As the trip wears on, I am tired and still need to recover from the jet lag. I excuse myself and retreat alone to my cot in the next cabin.

Not long after an attendant comes into the cabin. She says nothing but lowers and tightly closes the venetian blind on the window. Hmmm, I wonder what this all about. There must be something I am not permitted to see. Well now, my curiosity is aroused.

After she leaves, I sit by the window and pry apart ever so slightly the slats on the blind. As I peer through the slats, I see we are entering an area that looks like a city. Everything is concrete buildings. It is odd because I do not see any signs of life. There are no people, no cars or trucks, no activity on the streets, just an abandoned area of concrete structures. Even the fences and utility poles are concrete. I keep watch all through the area and the eerie sight never changes.

I later learned from John that this was a nuclear weapons depot and launch site for the former Soviet Union during the Cold War. I feel heavy at the thought that I have just seen an area that had nuclear weapons aimed at me only a few years ago. I am also relieved at the sight of it being an abandoned area.

As the day ends, I retire to my cot and try to sleep. Sleep comes slowly as I hear the never-ending clickity clack of the train traveling over the railroad track.

The next morning after 26 hours of train travel we transfer to a car and arrive at our destination in Ust'-Kamenogorsk. The weather in Almaty was spring like with the trees beginning to bud leaves in mid-April. Here it is still winter. There is still snow on the ground.

We travel immediately to a large dairy farm, formerly a Soviet communal dairy farm. It is very similar to the first farm we visited 26 hours south of here, near Almaty.

We meet the farm director, Vladimir, and his sons Peter and Igor. Vladimir is friendly but somewhat reserved. Peter stays in the background. Igor is outgoing, very friendly, and very inquisitive. He immediately attaches to me with a desire to learn whatever he can about me, my country, and the management of dairy cattle. It soon becomes evident to me that Igor is the one primarily overseeing the dairy cattle.

This is the farm for delivery of the ultrasound machine. I will show Igor how to use the ultrasound machine to diagnose pregnancies in dairy cows.

After a short tour of the farm, we immediately travel to one of the concrete dairy barns. Igor is anxious to see the ultrasound machine and learn how to use it. He is the main attraction in the barn. I notice that the barn personnel are at his beck and command. He is respectful and nice to them. They like him.

I assemble the machine and we start checking cows. These cows have not been checked for pregnancy for many months. I show Igor how to examine the cow and what to look for as a visual diagnosis of pregnancy on the ultrasound screen.

I become alarmed as cow after cow is not pregnant. There is a woman who has learned the technique of pregnancy diagnosis by palpation. She does not believe my open diagnosis.

She reaches into each cow I diagnose as non-pregnant and then backs away disappointed but in agreement.

I want to show Igor what a pregnancy looks like. I want him to see the heartbeat of the fetus. That is exciting. I check many cows for a long time and not one is pregnant. Finally I do find a pregnant cow and we spend a long time looking at it. Igor is insistent on formalizing that image in his mind. That is a good thing.

Less than a half dozen cows were pregnant that day after checking over a hundred. I say nothing but see the facial expressions of concern on Igor and his staff.

That evening I chat with Hisa, the man who organized our visit to these farms. I ask him why Igor wants the ultrasound machine. Hisa responds that Igor wants to be able to diagnose pregnancy at a stage earlier than 90 days as is the custom on his farm. I cringe and respond that I could easily teach him to make that diagnosis at 35 days without the ultrasound machine. Hisa responds with alarm that he did not know that was possible. He bashfully asks me to not mention that to Igor as we have gone to great lengths to deliver the ultrasound machine. Besides that, Igor is infatuated with the technology we have brought to his farm.

I finish this day with Igor. Our team is the recipient of an evening meal with his family. After a full day of gracious hospitality, we retire to a bunkhouse where I collapse from exhaustion and sleep well. There is no bathroom in the bunkhouse. Those primal urges require a cold snowy trip to an outhouse with no plumbing. I am thankful that John told me about carrying the small tissue packs.

The next day we visit other farms in the area. At each farm, we engage in discussions about issues important to them. I let them set the agenda. They are all very gracious and hospitable. Many of the farms are interested in nutrition. They understand that a dairy cow's work is converting fiber that is indigestible to humans into high-quality dairy foods and beef.

I use a computer program to show them predicted milk production from the feeds they offer their cows. The program predicts production close to their actual production. This gains their confidence in our discussions. I show them which nutrients are limiting the milk production of the cows on their farms. I show them what they need to do to improve the nutrition of the cows on their farms.

On all farms, I find that the limiting nutrient is protein. Each farm is an isolated unit that supplies all necessary feeds from their crops. They raise corn, barley, and grass hay. They harvest the corn as whole plant silage. They harvest the barley as grain. They harvest the grass as silage or dry hay. There is no supplemental protein source.

The cows are generally fat. They overfeed energy in the form of carbohydrates and under feed protein. The excess energy converts to fat. I need a supplemental protein source. In the U.S. we would use byproducts from other industries like soybean meal, canola meal, cottonseed meal, brewers grains, and the list goes on and on of available byproducts from other industries. None of these products are available. There are no feed mills to sell ingredients. Everything available to feed the cows grows on the farm.

I do notice that some farms grow a small amount of alfalfa. Alfalfa is a legume. Legumes pull nitrogen out of the air to produce a high protein forage. I conclude that if they cannot buy protein they need to grow it. I conclude by encouraging them to grow more alfalfa to feed their cows.

At the conclusion of each farm visit there is a meal served. It is the custom for the guest to offer a toast to their hosts. This is a former Russian country. Vodka is the beverage of choice. Shot glasses of vodka are always present. I offer a toast to my hosts for their health and prosperity on every farm. It is imperative to keep the shot glasses full to the brim. After several farm visits on the same day I soon realize that if I am to be coherent and of any informational use, I need to limit the volume of vodka I consume from these shot glasses. It seemed to be a game for them to challenge the guest to a contest. They would down shot after shot challenging me to do the same. I can only respond with "You win."

Some farms are of the Muslim faith. We sit on the floor or on short stools around a beautiful Persian rug stacked high with plates of vegetables, mutton, beef, and goat. It is custom for the guest to start the meal by biting off the ear of a roasted goat head and offer a toast of vodka to the hosts. I comply with a gracious smile and offer a toast through my interpreter.

After several days of these visits, it is time to return to Almaty on the train. On the day of our departure, Igor wants to spend more time with me with the ultrasound machine. I agree and we start checking cows again long before sun up and we do not quit until it is time to catch the train.

Our team boards the train in the nick of time before departure. The train has a standard loop it takes on every trip. That loop takes us across the border into Russia and the Siberian wilderness. We will travel further north before we turn around for the return trip to Almaty. It is a longer trip. I am exhausted. I hit the cot and fall asleep quickly.

A few hours later, I am rocked awake by a knock on the door followed by an uninvited entry to my room. Before me stands a Russian soldier glaring at me. My interpreter has possession of my travel documents and she assures me she would take care of all the legal and customs requirements. She is with the soldier. We are at the Russian border and the soldier insists upon seeing me. He asks me to stand and glares at me for a minute then leaves as abruptly as he came. I suspect that he just wanted to see what an American looks like. I am so sleepy and disheveled that I know it is not a pretty sight.

We return to Almaty and make a few more farm visits

similar to all the previous ones. On the final night before my departure, we hold a meeting of many local dairyman. They have become quite interested in raising alfalfa for their cows.

I speak with them about the benefits of providing more protein to their cows and how to harvest and store alfalfa silage. They are receptive to new information.

There was one man who was not buying it. He listened with a frown on his face. Finally, he stood up, introduced himself as Dimitri, demanded everyone's attention, and stated that he did not need any American advice on how to run his dairy. His dairy is just fine without American advice. He insisted that he could show the Americans a thing or two. Everyone else in the room ignored him and we continued with the meeting. Later Hisa told me to ignore the comment. That man has always been a problem and no one takes him seriously. On its best day his dairy is mediocre.

After the meeting, I say my goodbyes, pack my luggage, and travel to the Almaty airport. The trip back to the States is long. It will take thirty-six hours in planes and airports. On the final leg from London, I fall asleep after liftoff and I do not wake up until the plane is over Lake Michigan on the final descent into Chicago's O'Hare airport.

As I reflect on this experience, one observation that stands out to me is the receptivity of the vast majority of the people that I meet on the trip. Most are eager to gain information. All are curious about what I represent to them. They are not content to limit their understanding and knowledge to what they already possess. They desire to know and understand more.

Hisa has a passion to develop a new service industry where one currently does not exist. Igor finds technology unfamiliar to him to be a challenge. He is energetic in learning a new skill and applying it to his current circumstance. The presentation I give on my final night in the country leads to extensive questions and answers. People have within them an innate desire to gain new information. They desire to understand and apply that information to their lives.

Dimitri is the exception. His attitude is that he has nothing to learn. His mind is closed to everything beyond his self-imposed barriers and it appears that he will remain in that state. He may find himself left behind.

As time continues relentlessly onward so does the accumulation of knowledge gained by the curiosity and inquisitiveness of people. We possess this trait to a much greater degree than does any other species. No other species has invented a wheel, a car, a train, or an airplane. No other species has gone beyond visible light in the electromagnetic spectrum to invent radios, televisions, WIFI, cell phones, x-ray machines, and so much more.

More than any other species, people can choose to push themselves beyond the apparent barriers before them. They can choose to become familiar with the unfamiliar and make huge changes to their existence in a single lifetime. The challenge lies before each of us. We can be content to live our lives in a routine that focuses only on what we already know, or we can embrace a desire to investigate what we do not know.

CHAPTER 3

Unseen

"You can never reach the truth by
looking in the same direction all the time!"
— Mehmet Murat ildan

Today is Friday. I like Fridays. I can wrap up the workweek and look forward to the weekend. However, this weekend I am on call. This means that I will need to cover for any emergencies that come in from now until Monday. It is all part of my profession and it is a necessity.

It is 6 p.m. and all is quiet. A moment later, my cell phone lights up and delivers a text notification with its designated tune of "Who Let the Dogs Out?" I know what that means. It means I have an emergency call coming in from our Answering Service.

I reluctantly dig out my smartphone and read the new text. It reads: "Daniel has a cow off feed. C/B? Yes." He requests a phone call back to discuss his suspicions about this cow. I promptly place the call to Daniel. He is concerned about a sick cow. She refuses to eat her feed, her eyes are sunken, and she seems depressed. He wants me to come to his farm to examine the cow.

It takes about twenty minutes to drive to Daniel's farm. When I arrive, I follow my usual routine of putting on clean coveralls and boots and filling my trusty stainless steel bucket with warm water. This is the only bucket I have ever used on farm calls and it has survived many years of abuse. It carries a few scars from being kicked, trampled on, fallen on, or even driven over but it has always survived after some pounding and bending to restore its shape.

I meet Daniel in the barn and he leads me to the sick cow. I go through my usual routine of physical examination. First, I check her temperature. It is normal at 101.7. I place my stethoscope in my ears and listen on her left side for ruminations. Ruminations are the sounds one can hear as a cow's largest stomach contracts. They sound like the rumbling of thunder during a thunderstorm. The sounds build to a crescendo as the stomach contracts and then fade away as the stomach relaxes. Normally they occur about twice a minute. If they are not present, it often means the cow is not feeling well and has not been eating anything. As I listen, they are infrequent and weak.

Then I snap my finger against her skin over her left side while simultaneously listening with my stethoscope placed nearby. A ping sound occurs when the sound waves from the snap of one's finger against the skin of the cow travel through her tissues and reflect back to your stethoscope by a gas liquid interface. If one hears the reflected sound, or ping, it means there is an accumulation of gas in whatever structure lies beneath your stethoscope. I do not hear any pings anywhere on her left side.

I move forward to listen to her heart and lungs for abnormalities. I determine that her heart rate is elevated. This means she is enduring stress, pain, or dehydration. Now I move around to her right side and repeat many of the same examinations.

As I snap on her right side, I find a very large area that has a ping over most of her right abdomen and rib cage. I complete my exam checking for other possible conditions.

The large ping on the right side means that her fourth stomach, the abomasum, has an accumulation of gas within that causes the stomach to float upward along the right side of her abdomen. This is not the normal position in the lower abdomen. Because the stomach is not in a normal position, nothing can move through it. This creates an obstruction to the passage of contents and she refuses to eat her feed. As time passes, more gas accumulates within. The cow's condition and her prognosis continue to decline.

Daniel is waiting for my report. I inform him that his cow has a right displaced abomasum or as we say an RDA. This condition needs immediate surgical correction. If left uncorrected for too long the stomach will not recover function and the cow will die. It is Friday evening but this needs surgical correction now. He fully understands and agrees that I should go ahead with the surgery.

I go back to my car to retrieve my surgical supplies and return to the cow. She is standing in a stall.

As I go about my routine, I notice that a young boy is watching me. He appears to be about 9 years old. His eyes are bright, his hair is short, and he is intent on observing everything with an eagle eye on the details. He seems unusually confident in himself. He asks many questions as I proceed to prepare the cow for surgery. He asks who I am, what I am doing, and why the surgery is necessary. How long will it take? His name is Billy and he likes to talk. He tells me about his favorite cows and why he likes them. He tells me about his favorite jobs on the farm. He likes to help his dad do carpentry work. His dream is to be a carpenter when he grows up. He is already accumulating his own set of carpentry tools.

I keep my surgical supplies in a large toolbox made for carpenters. It has "Stanley," a maker of carpentry tools, written on the outside of the toolbox. Billy notices this toolbox and as his eyes light up with interest, he asks about it. "Why do you use that toolbox? Do you do carpentry work also?" I respond that I need to keep my instruments in something and yes I do some homeowner carpentry work around my house.

His eyes get larger. "So do you take all that stuff out of this box and put your carpentry tools in it when you do carpentry work? You need to keep your carpentry tools somewhere." I respond that I have another box for those tools.

I use hair clippers to remove the hair over a large portion of her right side. Then I scrub the surgical site with an iodine soap. I open my surgical kit, scrub my hands and arms, and don sterile latex gloves. Billy watches closely and keeps asking questions.

I take my sharp scalpel and make a deep diagonal incision about three inches behind the last rib. Blood oozes from the incision. Frankly, it gets a bit messy at this point with blood covering the area. Billy's eyes get even wider. I ask him if he has ever seen this before. I have had observers faint as they watch me make the incision. For the first time, Billy gets a little quiet and does not respond to my question.

I turn my attention back to the cow and continue my incision deeper into the abdominal cavity. Billy is quiet. I turn to check on him. He looks at the cow and then turns his attention to me. His eyes are big and round curious globes of puzzlement. Then out of the blue, Billy in a strong voice says this: "You know something Doc? You should stick with carpentry!"

I chuckle under my breath and say nothing. Billy watches the entire procedure with more questions and comments but none quite as penetrating as his comment encouraging me to stick with carpentry.

It is obvious to me that Billy can only see the visual aspect of the messy appearance of blood around the incision. He cannot see what lies beyond that appearance and the purpose of the surgery. He can only see the incision. He limits his understanding by his judgment of what is visible to him. He did not expand his understanding by looking for a reality beyond the visually obvious.

As I reflect on Billy, I realize that I can be like that myself. I think only about what I can see and what I know from my experiences. I often fail to look for a deeper reality beyond the obvious. I am preoccupied with my daily routine. I continue living on a day-by-day monotony, oblivious to anything else.

As my mind wanders into a place removed from the reality in front of me, I begin to ask questions of myself. What if there is a reality, a truth beyond the obvious, a supernatural place beyond this natural earth? If one reflects on the history of people, it is easy to observe that throughout our history people have constantly looked for just such a reality. The existence of anything beyond the obvious realities of our natural world seems ridiculous for much of our culture.

Yet big questions haunt us. Why is this planet such a special place that it can support life and the living as we know it? Why are people so much different than all other living things? What are intellect, emotions, dreams, visions, and ideas? Why have people been creative enough to invent things, cars, airplanes, computers, and much more? Why has no other species come even close to inventing things like we have? Where did I come from? Do I exist just to pursue personal pleasure and accumulate "Things?" Does my life have any particular purpose? What happens when I die? Should I be afraid of death? Is there anything beyond death? What does it mean when I read in the biblical book of Genesis that mankind was created in God's image?

Throughout the history of our species, we have sought answers to these questions. People developed societies, philosophies, and religions around their answers to these questions.

Native American cultures believe in harmony with themselves, their community, and their environment. Inherent in much of their beliefs is a strong recognition of a "Great Spirit" that has an all-encompassing power and that created all things. They conduct spiritual ceremonies and rites of life passages that recognize that this spirituality is not separate from their daily existence. These beliefs are their answer to the reason for their existence.

Ancient Greeks had an extensive tradition of gods and goddesses to describe the origin and nature of their lives and world. These mythical beings were immortal. They were ageless. They were the subject of art and literature. Temples were built and dedicated to them. They personified the origin of the world. They engaged in love, conflict, heroism, and tragedy. There were extensive descriptions of their activities and relationships in art and literature. They were considered divinities that influenced the lives of the people. These beliefs were their answer to the reason for their existence.

Ancient Egyptians developed a religion centered on animals and gods. These gods were to protect against chaos in their world. They were particularly concerned about the rising of the sun each day. The sun god, Re, would sail his boat under the world each night and defeat an evil spirit, Apophis, before he could rise again the next day. The gods also helped the dead into the next world that was better than the current world. They created many drawings and paintings in tombs and pyramids to honor their gods. They stocked their tombs with items they considered essential in the afterlife. The Pharaohs ruled over the people. The Pharaohs were considered divine. These beliefs were their answer to the reason for their existence.

Traditional African religions are diverse but share a common belief in multiple higher and lower gods. They involve a belief in spirits and respect for those who have passed on to another place. There is a focus on the "medicine man," healing, and magic. There is a belief that their ancestors are gods and they pray to them. There are religious ceremonies and rituals, often rhythmic with drums, to enhance a meditative state of mind. They believe in an afterlife in a spirit world.

Hinduism is the oldest religion. It encompasses a much larger number of beliefs and rules than other religions. They believe that every living creature has a soul and collectively they are all part of a supreme soul called "Parramatta." Human life aims to be one with this supreme soul and as such to experience Nirvana. Our lives consist of the good and bad things we do and this will determine our happiness in our next life. Our happiness in this life is a result of the good and bad we have done in previous lives.

Buddhists look internally to themselves to discover truths. Meditation is a big part of this religion. They seek Nirvana by looking within themselves for the truth or enlightenment of their life. They meditate to gain an inner stillness by sitting quietly in a serene environment to focus their awareness inward. It can also involve chanting, martial arts, or focusing on their breathing. They strive to lead a decent life that does not engage in killing living things. They speak kindly of others.

The Incas of the Andean mountains of South America worshiped nature. They had a mixture of ceremonies and beliefs in magical powers that culminated in worship of the sun. They had many gods of nature and astronomical constellations. They sacrificed both humans and animals on important occasions.

The Mayan religion of Central America was focused on creation. They paid a lot of attention to the cycles of their agriculture consisting of rain and harvest. Their gods were from nature and were important to them, the gods of the sun, rain, and corn. They, too, engaged in animal and human sacrifice.

Why have so many cultures throughout history engaged in a continuous quest to answer the big questions regarding the reason for their existence? Whether we know it or not we instinctively need to answer those big questions. Is there a reality beyond the obvious visual reality we see, hear, smell, taste, and feel every day? Is there such a thing as gods or a God? Why have cultures throughout history had a spiritual component? Why are there religions? Why are they controversial? Why have they continued to exist despite many attempts to abolish them? Why do they seem to get stronger when their very existence is challenged by persecution in an attempt to eliminate them? Why are there martyrs who give up their life for their belief in a spiritual reality? Why do most people have a reverence for the very existence of life? Why do many people have an innate desire to be helpful to others? This is certainly a noteworthy trait but not all people have that desire. Why do we even exist on this speck of dust called earth? Is it just happenstance? Is it just pure luck in the concurrence of astronomical events? Am I to believe that we are an accident, a chance happening among all of nature?

Alternatively, is there something else at play here? Could it be that there is an intentional aspect to our existence? Could it be that someone or something intended for humans to be unique among all other forms of life? Humans have been imagining a reality beyond the visually obvious throughout their existence in the form of traditions and religions. They have perceived and pursued a spiritual component to life. Humans seem to inherently know that someone or something intends their origin.

One may not place much credibility in the Bible as a book used for reference. Yet it is the greatest selling book of all time. Is that because mankind has an inkling to discover the truth about his origin and his intended purpose for existence?

Permit me to quote from this book. Genesis 1:27: "So God created mankind in his image, in the image of God he created them; male and female he created them." This was after God had created the universe, the planet, and all other living things. Then He created mankind in His image. So what does it mean that we are created in the image of God? God is in a much different reality from our physical existence. That reality, if it exists, is a timeless, infinite, beyond this earth's physical existence reality. That reality is not seen visually with the naked eye. It is not detected with a microscope, telescope, spectrophotometer, CAT scan, X-ray, multimeter, thermometer, NMR, or any other device designed to detect and analyze a physical object.

God is not of this world. He is a spiritual reality. He has created humans in His image meaning that we have a spiritual existence as well as a physical existence. If we do not believe that, then we will not perceive it and we will not discover it. However, if we at least consider it a possibility based upon the history of mankind's pursuit of such a reality, our lives will become an ever-increasing awareness of a spiritual reality. What drives some people to be good people and others to be bad people? Where does evil come from? Where do crimes against a person come from? What drives some people like Mother Teresa to devote their lives to benefit the poor and helpless among us and what drives others to harm people for their selfish indulgence? Good and evil exist. We cannot deny that. Yet we cannot measure it with a scientific instrument. Good and evil exist in that spiritual realm within us.

As humans, we all need to consider the possibility that there is a spiritual aspect to our lives. We need to consider that this is what it means to be created in God's image. That means there is a God.

When I deny the existence of God, what if I am wrong? Sooner or later, we all need to have answers to these questions. If we ignore them, we will wander in a sea of confusion. If we refuse to seek answers, we find ourselves in a life restricted to the accumulation of personal wealth and pleasures. If we limit our existence by only believing in what we can physically see, our lives will be nothing more than a legacy of selfish ambition.

We need to seek answers to these big questions. If we become seekers, we will live a life that endures trials and tribulations as well as the joys of living because we will find our value in what lies in the unseen.

CHAPTER 4

The Big Picture

"All that is made seems planless to the darkened mind,
because there are more plans than it looked for."

- C. S. Lewis, *Perelandra*

When a veterinarian finally receives their degree after the long years of schooling, they are excited to begin their new life as a veterinary doctor. Their first job is a new adventure for them but also challenging as they are aware of the need to prove their skills to their new clients as well as to themselves.

Our large animal veterinary practice has recently hired a new graduate from veterinary school. Her name is Kate. She comes to us with great credentials and we have confidence that she has a bright future. She is a hard worker, has a great young mind, and is excited to begin her career.

Not long after starting with us, Kate is excited to receive a call to examine a sick dairy cow on an Amish farm. She drives to the farm and parks her car alongside the barn.

Amos is the farm owner and operator. He is working his six-horse team in a field along the farm lane. As he sees Kate arrive at his farm, he, too, heads for the cow barn driving his team of horses to a resting area near the barn.

Draft horses are large and very strong. They are usually rather docile and mild mannered, cold blooded as we say. Their huge frame does demand respect as one well-placed kick from their rear legs or a strike from their front legs can kill a person. Their typical role on an Amish farm is to pull farm equipment through the fields. They just go about their duty to work hard, plowing on, monotonous mile after monotonous mile. They keep the status quo until they receive a command to do something different. They work together as a team.

There can be anywhere from one to six horses harnessed together pulling a farm implement. The workload determines the number of horses. There is a pecking order for the team of horses. A more experienced horse leads the team and the others obediently follow.

Kate is already in the cow barn. Amos quickly enters to lead her to the cow to examine. Kate starts her usual routine of physical examination of the cow, focusing on what is normal and what is not normal. She quietly takes the vitals and then places her stethoscope over the left side of the cow to listen for ruminations. All is quiet.

Suddenly there is a loud clatter outside the barn coming from the direction of the six-horse team. Kate and Amos are both alarmed and run to the door to see what the matter is.

Twenty-four feet are pounding the pavement outside the barn. The draft horse team has decided it is time to go back to work. As Amos emerges from the barn, he watches his team of horses clamber out the farm lane toward parts unknown, with no driver. Chasing them is fruitless as they are too far-gone and too fast to catch on foot.

Without thought, Amos does what comes naturally to him when driving his team. At the top of his lungs, he shouts "WHOA," a command for the horses to stop. The six-horse team, led by the lead horse, dutifully stop their adventure. They do an about-face and begin the trek back the long lane towards the barn.

Amos is thankful to see his workhorses galloping back towards the barns. As they near the buildings, the lead horse, by repetitive habit, goes directly towards the horse barn. The other five horses obediently follow alongside.

As the six-horse team approaches the barns, the leader runs along the right side of Kate's car. The other five have no choice but to follow the lead. Catastrophe is imminent.

There is not enough space for all of the horses to run alongside the car. These are big draft horses with thundering footsteps. Five pounding sets of four feet each, run up on the hood of the car, across the roof and down the back of the now demolished vehicle.

The horses are alarmed but unhurt. The five do exactly what they are trained to do. They dutifully follow the leader.

The lead horse is only aware of the circumstances that surround his immediate awareness. He is not aware of a bigger reality just beyond his perception. The remaining five occupy an unchanging existence of playing the game of follow the leader. They dare not challenge the status quo.

The life of a horse consists of their training, instincts, social relationships, and physical ability to perform mechanical work. That is their reality. They are aware of nothing else.

Ant colonies are well-organized social units comprised of individuals with specific duties united around a common purpose of sustenance, reproduction, and expansion of the colony. The queen lays eggs. The workers build and maintain the nest. The workers take care of the queen. The workers grow and gather food. They defend against their enemies.

Ants communicate with one other. They draw workmates to food sources. They unite to fight against an enemy. Their world consists of life within and around their colony. This is their only experience. Nothing else is real to them. Yet there is so much more life beyond their limited reality.

The same circumstances can seem familiar to the rudimentary existence of a person's life. Alternatively, people can search beyond those barriers with an innate capacity to discover new realities. People can discover a larger perspective of what may lie beyond that which is perceived with their biological sensory organs. That endeavor requires people to leave the status quo behind. They need to recognize their rudimentary plight. They need to desire to discover, to seek truth beyond the limitations of their biological and sociological existence.

People exist in communities united around a common purpose of survival, social experience, and reproduction. We interact with one another within the community. We interact with other communities, often friendly but sometimes violent. There are leaders and followers. Like the team of horses or the ant colony, we can find ourselves mired in a monotonous routine of existence, unaware of a greater reality beyond the visually obvious. What if there is a much larger reality to discover if one engages the effort to find it? What if we never find it because we did not take the effort to seek it? Just as the lead horse returning to Amos' barn is only aware of the consequences of his own experience, we may limit ourselves to the boundaries of our personal experience.

Our species is quite unique in that we possess a higher capacity to investigate our interests. We seek to learn what makes things work. We have been on an ever-expanding accumulation of knowledge that includes the tiny unseen details of microscopic life to the expanse of the infinite universe. We have a desire to learn more about our existence.

Consider the mass expanse of the universe and the complexity of life on this one little speck of dust called earth. Is this planet and the life on it the result of statistical probability? Can it be that if we draw on our capacity to be curious that we can discover a reality beyond the boundaries of this natural existence?

We believe that life came into existence by evolving through a parade of biochemical interactions resulting in a variety of life forms that survive in a hostile environment. Those best suited to survive reproduce their DNA to continue the timeline of life. The best-adapted species continue to produce the variety of current life forms on this planet. The less suited to survive species are overcome by their inadequacies and disappear.

Contrast that with the belief that an intelligent creator planned the formation of life. Can it be that the continual production of variety within a species is part of a master plan? Can it be that survival of the fittest, those best adapted in that sea of a variety of life forms, are part of a master plan? Can it be that those life forms that are at a distinct disadvantage and cease to survive are part of a master plan?

Humankind has instinctively sought after a spiritual reality throughout history. It is a reality beyond the visually obvious. The creator is God who had a master plan to make an environment suitable for life. He placed life forms in that environment to interact with one another in a carefully engineered manner that propagates life in its many forms on this planet.

He did this to produce an advanced life form where every individual would draw upon their abilities to discover Him, to honor Him, to worship Him, and to be in a constant relationship with Him. God desires companionship with that which He created and He placed that desire for companionship within humans.

These two belief systems seem to be a contradiction. Our society tells us we must adhere to one or to the other. One cannot believe both.

I struggled with knowing which to claim as my belief. I like science. I like to understand how things work. The scientific method is a protocol to determine truth. It is based upon our ability to investigate an idea with a rational approach that limits bias. I cannot throw science out the door to claim an alternative belief not based upon reason. Science is our quest to understand the world around us. As time passes that understanding becomes better, but it never reaches completeness.

We do not have a complete understanding of all that encompasses the reality before us. We have made a lot of progress going from the invention of the wheel to interplanetary travel, not to mention all the other things we have invented and mass-produced to make our lives more comfortable. We still do not know it all and I do not believe we ever will have a full understanding in this present life.

I personally have also experienced many revelations from God that bring me to a place where I cannot deny His existence. I am confused by two opposing belief systems. On one hand there is a scientific explanation based upon observations and a rational explanation for the existence of life. On the other hand, I am intrigued by the instinctive pursuit of a spiritual truth. I am caught between an undeniable belief in a God who created life and a science that offered an alternative rational explanation absent of an intelligent creator. However, there can only be one truth. The two must be one.

Perhaps that is the key to resolving this conflict. Some assume that since God did not explain the details of how He created life, the origin of the universe and of life must have been some process beyond reason, beyond science. Assumptions can lead us astray. The scientific method is designed to either validate theories or discredit them. I cannot deny that there is variability between individuals and populations within species. I cannot deny that natural selection and survival of the fittest occur. These forces describe how a species adapts to a changing environment. Those best adapted will survive and reproduce. Those species unable to adapt will disappear.

Perhaps the forces we know as evolution are in some part the mechanism by which God created. Do those two concepts need to be opposed to one another? We cannot fuse the two into truth because our knowledge is incomplete.

Truth is truth regardless of whether it came through scientific discovery or from revelation by God. Unlike the team of horses and the ant colony, humans are capable of escaping the monotony of a routine existence through their capacity to investigate the unknown. We should endeavor to resolve these conflicts in order to come to a better understanding of origin and purpose.

CHAPTER 5

Coincidence?

"The probability of a certain set of circumstances coming together in a meaningful (or tragic) way is so low that it simply cannot be considered mere coincidence."

— V. C. King

Veterinary school is a challenging endeavor for every student. The early years demand a total commitment to long hours of lectures, laboratory work, and outside the classroom study. Students are told to spend three hours of time studying outside of class for every hour in the classroom.

I started my veterinary schooling with apprehension of my ability to meet the demands of effort and time required to be successful. One is subconsciously aware of their self-doubt for much of that first semester. It is not until one has success in their first set of final exams that they begin to develop confidence that "I can do this."

It is Sunday evening of the final weekend of my first semester. Christmas is less than three weeks away. Final exams begin tomorrow on Monday. I have spent the entire weekend preparing for final exams. I leave my books for a moment to take a break with Joyce. We both need a break from the apartment. A thought simultaneously pops into both of our heads. Let us go back to my parents' farm to retrieve some Christmas decorations for our tiny apartment. We need to cheer the place up a bit.

On the spur of the moment, Joyce and I put on our winter coats and head out the door. We start up our trusty navy blue Volkswagen bug and embark on the hour-long drive to the farm. We chat cheerfully along the way, just glad for the welcome break.

As we drive on the small road that borders the farm, we notice a neighbor's car parked along the shoulder of the road near the barn. That is an odd place to park a car. We ignore it thinking they must have had car trouble. Maybe we can help them.

I drive the car into the driveway and park by the house. As we both open the doors to exit the car, the neighbor lady comes running to meet us. The first words from her mouth are "God must have sent you here right at this time."

She hurriedly explains that she was driving on the road near our barn when my mother came running out to the road to flag her down because she needed help. My mother was distraught and did not know what to do. My mother had just discovered my father lying on the ground in the pen where we kept a bull. She had gone to find him because he never came in from the barn to eat supper with her. She saw the car on the road and ran for help. The car's occupant is our neighbor who immediately calls for an ambulance. Joyce and I arrive just moments later before the ambulance arrives.

Without thought and not wanting to believe what I just learned, I run to the bullpen to see for myself. I find my father lying motionless on the ground. His condition is obvious. There are no signs of life. One never forgets this visual image. It is as clear to me now as it was many years ago. The emotion fades but the image does not fade. This is an abrupt change to my life. Until this happened I felt that bad things only happened to other people. Now it is real for Joyce and myself. Bad things can happen to anybody.

I spend the next few hours making phone calls to my

brothers, friends, and extended family. Some of them come to our assistance this same evening even though it is getting late. It is comforting to have family and close friends nearby.

Joyce and I stay at the farm. We try to sleep. It does not happen. I toss and turn the entire night. What does this mean for Joyce and I and our immediate future?

My father sold the mature cows a month before I went to veterinary school. After I left it was just mom and dad tending to the farm. My oldest brother still lived on the farm but held a full-time job off the farm. He is not home much. My other brother lives in New York City where he is busy with his schooling and a full-time job. There are still heifers remaining on the farm. They need to be cared for. My mother is alone. My final exams begin tomorrow morning. Should I quit veterinary school? That would seem to be the reasonable thing to do.

The next morning Joyce and I travel back to our apartment to retrieve clothing as we only had those that were on our backs. Our emotions are at full steam. At one point, I pull off the road and my emotions burst forth. Joyce is there for me. I sob on her shoulder.

I call the veterinary school to explain what has happened and that I will not be coming back to school this week to take final exams. They are very understanding. They tell me to take as much time as I need. They tell me this is not the time to make hasty decisions.

The week that follows is filled with funeral planning, the funeral itself, and deciding what to do with the immediate demands of the farm. I am torn. I love the farm. I have also worked very hard to be admitted to veterinary school.

If it were not for my father who unselfishly encouraged me to continue pursuing my dream, I never would have been admitted to the school. Many farm families desire to pass on the farm to their next generation. I was the only one still available to stay on the farm. Yet my father encouraged me to pursue another dream. It seemed like it was part of his dream for me as well.

Joyce and I decide to try to make everything work out. I will stay in veterinary school and at the same time provide as much support to the farm as I am capable. This means traveling to the farm on weekends. I will provide the support needed for my mother to feed the cattle during the week. It means support from my brothers as much as they are able. My mother will feed the cattle during the week and Joyce and I will stay at the farm on weekends. I will spend my summer vacation from school operating the farm.

There are still final exams to take. In my shaken frame of mind and with my self-doubt, I am not confident of a positive outcome. I arrange to take the exams over the Christmas break. I meet with the professors and they support my decision and agree to administer the exams. The exams are in the form of essay answers to questions. I like this format because it allows me to write the answers as I know them. I will not need to decipher an obscure answer to a trick question. Just tell them what you know. I take the exams and I pass all of them. This is a boost to my decision and to my confidence.

Coincidence is defined as a striking occurrence of two or more events at one time apparently by mere chance. Four events occurred almost simultaneously on that Sunday evening. First, Joyce and I make a rash decision to travel to the farm. Second, while we are traveling to the farm, my mother decides to go look for my father. Third, as she finds him, my neighbor drives by on the road to coincide with my mother's rush to the road, in a panic, to seek help. Fourth, moments later Joyce and I arrive on the scene before the ambulance arrives.

Could all four events be a coincidence? I suppose they could be if I am determined to believe that they are a coincidence. However, there comes a point where it is more rational to believe otherwise. These four events timed so closely together at just the right moment to ease the trauma to my mother seem to have been arranged by a higher power. One then must begin to examine the possibility of a reality beyond the visually obvious.

Christianity as a religion has alienated many people by its focus on a set of rules and rituals that vary between different groups. They see rules that are irrelevant and rules that are ridiculous. The rituals appear to celebrate nothing more than historical events. To find meaning and purpose for their life, people take pride in being their own person. They take pride in forging their own path through life. They do not need a religious crutch to lean on.

Setting aside the distraction of the superficial aspects of religion, the core issue that comes before everyone sooner or later is a need to discover if it is possible that there is a spiritual reality beyond our very physical lives. Forget about the rules and rituals. Many of those are constructed by human minds. Humans are fallible. Instead, search for a truth where the grass grows greener that lies beyond the boundaries of our physical existence.

CHAPTER 6

Defeating the Giants

*"We are not human beings having a spiritual experience.
We are spiritual beings having a human experience."*
- Pierre Teilhard de Chardin

The 2018 World Cup Soccer Tournament featured the world's best soccer teams from countries that had competed in preliminary games to be part of the World Cup games. The tournament featured the usual elite teams representing countries like Great Britain, France, Spain, Germany, Brazil, Mexico, Argentina, Portugal, and many more.

Germany was the favored team to dominate the games and had earned that reputation as a winner of the last World Cup in 2014.

Preceding the World Cup tournament, teams play one another worldwide to qualify for play in the World Cup. Germany dominated the teams they played and qualified for the 2018 World Cup as a favorite to win all the way through to the final championship game.

In the opening round of the tournament, Germany came upon some intense competition. By the final game of the first round of play, they found themselves in need of a win to qualify for the next level of play in the tournament. The team they were to play and against which they needed a win was from South Korea. By all analysis, it should be an easy game for them to dominate and win. Media personnel announced that it should be an easy win for Germany. There were assured of advancing to the next round of tournament play.

The South Korean coach told his team before the game that he would give his own team a one percent chance of winning the game. South Korea had nothing to play for as they had already fared poorly and been eliminated from advancing to the next round of play in the tournament. Any reasonable person could see that this game meant nothing to the South Koreans, and it was life or death to the Germans. The German team had to play well and get the win.

As the game gets under way, the South Koreans rise to the challenge. Their players play beyond their ability against a bigger, better, more experienced German team. The Germans dominate the game. At halftime, the score is still an unexpected scoreless tie.

As the second half resumes, the South Koreans come out strong and persistent against the frustrated Germans who outshot the South Koreans 28 to 12. Many of the German shots are high and wide of the goal. The shots that are on target are saved by the South Korean goalkeeper.

As the game continues, the South Koreans pick up their level of play even more. They play beyond everyone's expectations. The German frustration grows. They are unable to score. At the end of regulation play, the score is 0-0. It appears that the game is heading toward penalty shots to determine the winner.

In added time for injury during the 92nd minute, the South Koreans were able to score and take a 1-0 lead in the game. The Germans are frantic. They must win this game or be eliminated in the early round of the World Cup.

The German goalkeeper leaves his goal box and becomes an added field player to bolster the German attack on South Korea. The goalkeeper gains position of the ball at midfield. The South Korean forward challenges him for the ball and strips the ball from the German attack. The South Korean scores an additional goal in the empty German net. South Korea wins the game 2-0.

In the history of the World Cup, the mighty German teams have not been eliminated during the first round of play since 1938. They are devastated. The South Koreans are ecstatic.

What is it in the human experience that inspires a person, or in this case a team to rise far above expectations? Their actions exceed rational explanation because there is a spirit within them that drives them to excellence. This is evidence of a spiritual reality and power beyond mere existence. Throughout history, humans have instinctively sought for a spiritual reality.

Click back in time to the biblical story of David vs. Goliath. David the shepherd boy has no armor. His only weapon is a primitive slingshot. He is confronted with the mighty Goliath towering over him in full armor and weaponry. Yet little David volunteered to fight the giant. All reason would say it is not a match David can win. He will lose his life in an instant.

David's years as a shepherd boy watching his father's sheep prepared him for such a moment. He is alone out in the fields watching over the sheep. It is a boring job day after boring day. As a little boy with idle time, he finds ways to entertain himself. He picks up a leather strap. He finds some flat round stones and challenges himself to sling the stones at targets before him. Day after day, he slings the stones at various targets. He hits rocks. He hits clumps of grass. He increases the distance to the target. With much repetitive practice, he is good with the slingshot. He is very good.

His passion is protecting the vulnerable sheep he watches for his father. He kills lions and bears to protect the flock. His confidence improves with each success. He is possessed with a desire to excel. It has become part of his identity. He is following a drive that is within himself. He is unaware that he is preparing for a greater, divine event.

Now he sees the mighty Goliath from a safe distance. He remembers his experiences protecting the flock of sheep. He sees a way to confront the mighty giant. Goliath is in full armor. David has no armor. Yet there is a gap in the armor plates on Goliath's forehead.

The spirit within David drives him onward with confidence that is greater than fear. Spiritual leading has prepared him for this challenge. He picks up a few stones. He examines them. This one is perfect. He loads the slingshot. He whirls it around and around. He fires from a safe distance beyond the reach of the mighty Goliath. The sharp stone lands perfectly between the armor plates on Goliath's head. Goliath is surprised and stunned. He falls to the ground. David uses Goliath's own weapon to complete the task. Goliath is dead.

There is a spiritual reality within each person. It can inspire us to perform beyond our natural ability. It can guide us beyond our ability to reason. It can be used for good or for evil. The choice of the spirit we follow is ours. The reality of the spirit is not our choice, only our response to the spiritual leadings within. We can suppress them, ignore them, or listen to them.

As followers of Christ, we have within us the Spirit of Jesus that will always have our best interests at bay in spite of ourselves. When we have giants to face in our daily walk, the Holy Spirit is within us, available to guide us through that battle with confidence that our ultimate good is His intent.

However, the Holy Spirit will not impose His will upon us. We need to first discern Him then walk into the battle with courage and the confidence that He has already prepared us for the challenge, just as God had prepared little David for Goliath. The courage and confidence come from knowing that God has a master plan for each life. It is sometimes within and sometimes beyond our human reason.

Know that there is a spiritual world of reality beyond our

natural experience. Know that with the guidance of the Holy Spirit you can face the giants with courage and defeat them. It does not mean life will be easy. It does not mean the giants in our life must disappear. However, it does change our attitude so that the giants are not so big after all. Because it teaches us to grow in our faith, courage, and confidence. God has our back for our long-term best interests, especially when we cannot grasp the long-term consequence.

The giant that we often face may be a giant within us. It is our pride in our own ability to understand reality. Inherently we believe only in what our five senses bring to us. We are born with these boundaries. They are a giant obstacle to discovering a spiritual reality. Yet humans have instinctively sought after such a reality.

There is a spirit within us that is not contained by our biological senses. It inspires us to overcome that giant of pride in ourselves. It inspires us to always learn more, to investigate the unknown. To do so we must be willing to tackle the obstacles of self-pride, peer pressure, and apathy.

Pierre Teilhard de Chardin was a French Jesuit priest, scientist, and paleontologist. He served as a stretcher-bearer during World War I. During those years, he developed his reflections and recorded them in diaries and letters. One famous quote of his is: "We are not human beings having a spiritual experience. We are spiritual beings having a human experience."

CHAPTER 7

Determination

*"You do not really understand something
unless you can explain it to your grandmother."*
                                        - Albert Einstein

I t is a warm and pleasant mid-summer day, a perfect day for a bike ride on a delightful rail trail nearby. Joyce and I decide to do the ride. The trail along the Susquehanna River offers a variety of landscapes through forests, farmland, abandoned canals, and riverbank scenes. We enjoy the ride and return to our home.

As we open the back door to enter our house, our golden doodle dog, Jake, meets us. He bolts through the open door and circles the house barking ferociously while gazing upwards at our roof. Jake is a comical dog. He makes us laugh. This behavior is common. He will act as though he is protecting us but he is a coward. He soon settles down and comes back into the house.

As I take a quick glance out of the window, I notice a very large and somewhat cumbersome bird fly from the roof of the house and land on the driveway beside the house. Joyce sees it, too, and we both note that it is a peacock. It must have come from the farm across the road and we decide that it will find its way back home. Peacocks are not migratory birds and do not travel great distances. They are beautiful birds. Great intellect does not necessarily accompany great beauty. Their brain is not much larger than a pea and their powers of reasoning are primitive at best. We will give it some time to return to its home.

The next morning is a new day and I start this day as I do most days. I answer incoming phone calls for our veterinary business. Most are calls requesting our services for dairy cattle. At 8 a.m. it is routine for me to call my business partner, Bridget, to discuss the work for the day and split up the calls among our staff.

As I speak with Bridget, I also half-jokingly ask if she is missing a peacock. I know she has a pair of peacocks (Jack and Jill) in her barn. Bridget lives about three miles from my house. I am sure that it is not her peacock as that is too far away.

Surprisingly she says that her female peacock, Jill, has been missing for two weeks. My suspicion is aroused. Was our peacock sighting yesterday her peacock named Jill? I tell her about the experience yesterday afternoon with Jake and the peacock on our house roof. She thought I was joking and she did not believe me.

It took me quite a bit of persuasion to convince her that I did see a peacock on my house roof. I was sure it was not Jill because it is too far from her house and it would seem very unlikely for her missing peacock to show up on the roof of my house. Even if that is true, it is unlikely for the peacock to be seen by us again because Jake had scouted the place last evening for intruders and driven them away. The peacock has surely moved on to another location.

That afternoon, Bridget comes to our veterinary office with a large blue net. She insists on coming to my house. She is going to pursue finding and capturing the peacock. She asks if I would show her where I last saw the peacock.

Success in this endeavor seems unlikely to me. I doubt that the peacock is still at or near my house.

Bridget insists on giving it a chance. If we do not try, we

will surely fail. Success belongs to those willing to tackle a task that seems impossible.

Ok, I agree with that. Besides, this will be entertaining. If we find the bird, it will be two veterinarians chasing a peacock through the neighborhood in July heat of 90 plus degrees trying to capture the peacock with a net. I hope we will not be a feature article in the local newspaper.

The first order of business is to leave Jake in the house. Then we walk slowly and quietly around my property glancing broadly for any sign of the peacock. There is no sign of the bird.

We broaden our search as we walk across my neighbor's yard. Than we search beyond that onto the next neighbor's yard. I am becoming a bit apprehensive about venturing onto his yard. This is the neighbor that my kids affectionately call "The Mean Man." In their neighborhood play, they sometimes venture too close to his property. This guy will grump at them and tell them to stay away from his property. He is grumpy and not friendly towards them.

I express my misgivings to Bridget. She is undeterred. Her focus is on one objective—finding the bird. Therefore, she leads the way onward and we trespass on the "Mean Man's" property.

There is an old pickup truck in the driveway. I take a quick peek under the truck. Much to my surprise, I see a beautiful peacock resting quietly under the truck. I cannot believe it. The bird is still in the neighborhood. I look again, just to be sure. It is definitely the peacock.

Bridget is not far away. I quietly call for her to come to the other side of the truck informing her that we have found the bird. Perhaps I can push the bird away from me towards her where she can catch it with the net. The chase begins.

Bridget crouches down alongside a rusty wheel on the other side of the truck. She is ready to snag the bird. I begin to crawl under the truck towards the bird. Jill responds by retreating away from me and towards Bridget. Just a few more steps and Jill will be in the net. As Jill emerges from under the truck, Bridget swings the net in a swooping arc. Just as the net begins to surround Jill, she dodges to the left and escapes. This is not going to be as easy as we expected it to be.

Jill runs for her life into the wooded area behind the "Mean Man's" house with Bridget and myself on either side of her running in close pursuit. We find ourselves in an area cluttered with old abandoned cars, lawn mowers, furniture, discarded building materials, and other items that have accumulated behind the "Mean Man's" house over his lifetime.

All these obstacles are grown over with vines and weeds that make for difficult pursuit of Jill. We dodge trees, junk, and vines. Jill has plenty of opportunity to lodge beyond our reach. Every time we try to surround her, she dodges on to another hiding place.

For the next hour, we chase Jill through the woods and back and forth across the "Mean Man's" property. At long last, we have her cornered in a tight spot where she cannot escape. Bridget closes in on Jill for the catch. Just as she swings the net, Jill takes to the air and flies up high onto the roof of the "Mean Man's" house.

Bridget remains determined and focused on one goal, catching the peacock. No one has emerged from the house even though we are trespassing on the property. We have not yet been the target of the "Mean Man's" ire.

I reluctantly follow Bridget's lead towards the house. We can hear a loud radio sounding from inside the house. Someone must be at home in the house. I decide to be proactive and so I knock on the "Mean Man's" door. Perhaps if I explain our predicament he will allow us to continue our pursuit of Jill.

As I approach the house door, I notice a sign posted above the back door. It proclaims the residence to be "REDNECK ALLEY." Bridget asked if I thought he had guns. I respond that I would assume that he does.

I knock boldly on the "REDNECK ALLEY" door. There is no answer. I knock again, even louder. No one comes to the door. It seems there is no one home. Conversely, they may be taking a long nap and have the radio on as a distraction to other noises.

Meanwhile, Jill is resting from her flight up on the "Mean Man's" house roof. Bridget decides to climb up on the roof. She sees that she can climb up a tree at the back of the house onto a porch roof above the "Red Neck Alley" sign and from there climb onto the house roof. She successfully makes the climb. I hand her the net.

The radio in the house is playing John Denver's "Take Me Home, Country Road." Bridget begins her trek over the "Mean Man's" house roof. I take up a position in front of the house to watch her determined pursuit of Jill.

Peacocks like high places. Jill is perched on the top of the house roof. She watches as Bridget approaches. As Bridget crawls up the roof, Jill nonchalantly leaves her perch and flies back down to the yard on the side of the house. Bridget is unfazed. She climbs down from the roof. Once again, we chase Jill through the thicket behind the house. There is still no response from the residence.

Jill is weary of the unwelcome attention. She abandons the "Mean Man's" property and runs across the lawns towards my house. Looking for safe shelter, she runs into the wooded area beside my house.

This time we are not in close pursuit. We look for Jill but cannot find her. We did see her enter the wooded area but we do not know where she went after entering the woods. Bridget is still of single-minded determination to capture Jill. She is unwavering in her commitment to the task.

The net is not working. We need to change our strategy. It is time to develop a new plan. Jill is tiring and looking for safe shelter. Perhaps we can herd her into my garage.

Sometimes peacocks like shiny things. A farm we service has peacocks. On several occasions, I have noticed a peacock perched on top of the milk truck on the shiny milk tank. I open my sliding garage door. Inside the garage is a shiny bright orange tractor. Perhaps she will be attracted to the shiny tractor. If we can entice her into the garage and then shut the door, we will have her where she cannot escape.

We have a new plan. However, we have lost sight of Jill. We last saw her wander into the woods beside my house. Bridget and I slowly and quietly walk into the wooded area to locate Jill. After a brief unproductive search, Jill escapes from her hiding place in a thicket and startles us. She hurriedly runs across my lawn towards the garage. I hope that she has had enough of our persistent pursuit. I hope that she looks for safe shelter.

Jill runs towards the garage. We follow at a distance so as not to distract her attention. She continues towards the garage, enters through the open door, and darts to safety under the shiny orange tractor.

We follow and carefully slide the door closed. Finally, after a long and determined chase we caught Jill inside my garage. Bridget returned Jill to her rightful home and reunited her with Jack, her companion peacock. It is a happy ending and reward for determined persistence to accomplish a goal.

People have the ability to look beyond their mundane existence to achieve a better circumstance. They can have the awareness that they do not need to accept what may seem to be inevitable. People have within them the capacity to focus single-mindedly on a goal, if they choose to persistently seek that outcome. Just as Bridget was determined to pursue the peacock, people can be determined to seek answers to questions that fill their minds.

At some point, we wonder about the miracle of life that surrounds us. We question if there is a purpose for our lives beyond our mere existence. We can become complacent and not search for answers. That attitude can lead to a depressing life unfocused and without purpose. Alternatively, we can determine that our life purpose is to make the lives of those around us better. That is desirable and honorable, but it still does not answer the big question of why do we exist.

Conversely, we can become determined to search for a higher purpose beyond our own paradigm. We can shed our reservations about searching for what may seem to be unsearchable. Seek and ye shall find. It starts with seeking. Without seeking, there is no finding. With lifelong persistence, we will find answers.

Imagine what our lives could become if, like Bridget's pursuit of the peacock, we were so focused on finding God that we did not waiver from that purpose. We choose to ignore the distractions around us. As we search for God, we see Him in unexpected ways. It may be far different than our preconceived notions about a judgmental God that spoils our fun.

We may find a God that ultimately provides our best interests beyond what we expect. We may discover the meaning of grace, unconditional love, and unmerited favor. We may find an undeniable peace within ourselves that dispels the fears and disappointments that surround us. We may find a freedom from our own self-imposed rules that defy a subtle peace within our soul.

We may find a God that does not impose His will upon us but rather allows us the freedom to choose Him or to leave Him. It takes determination to find answers. It takes effort to go beyond our apathy to reach a place of confidence. We do not understand our own position unless we expend the effort to discover truth.

CHAPTER 8

Big Loving John

"Never lose an opportunity of seeing anything beautiful, for beauty is God's handwriting."
- Ralph Waldo Emerson

It is a rainy Sunday afternoon. I receive a call from John to come quickly to his farm. He has a Hereford cow that is having difficulty delivering a calf. She needs help. He is frantic. Please come right away.

I rise from my Sunday afternoon slumber and drive to his farm. I know the location of his farm but I have not been there previously. The farm is along a road I travel often.

The buildings are in an obvious state of disrepair. The barn is a typical style bank barn like many others in this area. The barn has massive stone walls as a foundation and has limestone walls on both ends of the structure. The stone in these thick walls is laid by masons skillfully arranging irregular shapes of stones from surrounding fields like a gigantic jigsaw puzzle. The walls on the sides of the barn are framed and sided with wood and then painted red.

The barn has two levels. The bottom floor is suitable for housing animals. It has pens and troughs for feeding and watering the animals. Above this ground level floor is a second level that is suitable for storing feed for the animals below. There are large areas for storing hay and grains for feed and straw for bedding the stalls below. The back of the barn has a ramp of dirt that rises from ground level to provide access to the second floor. Hence the name "bank barn." John's bank barn needs repairs and desperately needs a fresh coat of red paint.

I arrive at the farm and as is my usual custom drive to a door leading to the lower level of the barn and park my vehicle where I will have easy access from the barn. I expect to find John anxiously coming to meet me so that he can show me the way to the Hereford cow in need of calving assistance. I see no one. I wait a few minutes, but still see no one. I do not know if the cow is in the barn or out in the pasture behind the barn. I need to find John.

John's house is nearby. Like the barn, it too is in a state of disrepair. His house has endured many years of weather. I decide to walk to the house to see if I can find John. I walk upon the broken slabs of concrete that form the sidewalk. They lead me to a side porch of the house. I notice an old dog lying beside the house. The dog is a friendly Labrador retriever that apparently has seen many years of life. Too lazy to rise, the dog wags his tail as a friendly greeting.

As I reach the steps leading to the side porch, I can see more closely the condition of the house. Shutters on the house are broken. Wild vines are growing everywhere. A well-kept house should have flowers and shrubbery.

The wooden porch floor has broken and rotting boards. Some of the wooden steps are rotten and broken. I place my feet carefully only on the steps that appear to be able to support me. I carefully walk across broken boards to the door of the house. There is a screen door sagging from one hinge. The solid wooden door behind it needs repair and paint.

There are still no signs of John. I knock on the door and wait. There is no answer. I knock again, a little louder and wait. There is still no answer. I know he must be somewhere on the farm. Before I leave the house, I want to be certain that John is not in the house. I knock very loudly on the door.

As I turn to leave, the door slowly creaks open. There stands John. His shoulders slump over a large frame that shows the wrath of many years of labor on the farm. His face displays the ravages of years working in the sun. His wrinkles have wrinkles. He wears a slight smile of relief to see me. He speaks loudly to greet me.

We walk slowly to the barn. John is quiet. I stir up friendly conversation. We enter the lower level of the barn through a half-rotten Dutch door and walk down a long alley to a box stall at the other end of the barn. As I peer into the stall, I see a cow lying down on her side and groaning with every involuntary push that came to her. The stall is dirty with areas of manure that have accumulated with her activity in the stall. As we both enter the stall, the large Hereford cow stands up and puts her head in a corner away from us.

I begin my examination of the cow. A normal delivery presents the calf front feet and head first. They literally dive from their home of the past 280 days. I determine that the calf is coming with its head turned back. This is not normal and is preventing a normal delivery. I work to bring the head to a proper position. I notice that I do not feel any movement of the calf. I place my finger in its mouth to elicit a suckling reflex and there is no movement. These signs would seem to indicate that the calf is no longer alive.

As I work "Big John" frequently asks me if everything is going to be OK. I sense his great concern. Sometimes the calf is alive even though I do not elicit any reflexes during delivery. I simply reply with a smile and reassure him that I will do everything I can for both cow and calf.

I get both front feet and the head in the proper position so that I can deliver the calf. The cow continues to push and now that the presentation is normal, she makes continual progress with each contraction. With minimal assistance, the calf enters the outside world. I gently assist the calf to the floor of the stall behind me. I check for signs of life. There is no eye reflex. There is no breathing. There is no heartbeat. In spite of these dismal signs, I try to revive it but I am unsuccessful. The calf is deceased.

I turn away from the calf lying on the floor behind me and focus my attention back to the cow. I always check for a second twin calf. I check for damaged tissues from the delivery.

As I focus my attention on the cow, I hear activity behind me. Out of the corner of my eye, I become aware of John behind me. As I turn my attention to the activity behind me, I see Big John sitting down amid the manure-covered floor of the stall. He has gathered up the deceased calf in his arms. He is hugging it. Tears are streaming down his face. He is crying. He is distraught. His quiet moans touch my heart. It is evident to me that he has lost an expected beloved member of his family.

I deliver a lot of calves. Death is part of life. Sometimes the calf does not survive a difficult delivery. One can become hard and insensitive to that outcome. It is easy for me to be rather mechanical in my actions and attitudes. I distance my feelings from that loss of life.

Seeing Big John's response to the deceased calf convicts me that I have not responded with compassion. I am convicted of my hardness. Big John is an introvert. He lives alone. He chooses to be apart from most people. He is elderly. His cows and his calves are his family. They are what energize him and give him a reason to live. He cares deeply for them. He has just suffered the loss of a family member. He is their father and he loves them dearly. They depend on him for the provision of their needs of shelter, food, water, and protection.

As I reflect on this experience with "Big John," I am drawn into contemplating the meaning of love. Big John loves his family of cattle. To him, these cattle are more than just residents of his farm. He loves them. He knows them individually. He has a relationship with them. They provide companionship for him.

In a rudimentary form, love is a part of much of the animal kingdom. When a cow delivers a calf, she turns and instinctively begins caring for the calf. If she did not care for the calf, it would die. Love is like a spiritual magnet. When you love someone, you are drawn to them. You want to see them more often. You desire to spend time with them. You want to know more about them. You want to understand them. You want to protect them. You do not force your way upon them, but rather allow them freedom to make choices. They are not slaves. They are companions.

Our bodies, like much of the animal kingdom, have a basic set of physical characteristics. Our bodies consist of a core that contains the organs necessary to sustain life, surrounded by four appendages and a tail to provide for locomotion, balance, and the ability to grasp and maneuver things. At the top of the body is a control center to coordinate all activities.

However, there is no organ in our bodies called love. It is an aspect beyond the physical composition of our bodies. Yet love is so much a part of our lives. It is the opposite of hate. Both love and hate are wrapped around our personal relationships. They influence our responses within those relationships. Both are evidence of a spiritual reality within us.

I think of Big John sitting in a pile of manure. He is cradling and hugging tightly his wet, deceased calf. It gives me a mental picture of how deep God's love is for His people. He loves us no matter what condition we are in, no matter where we are, no matter what we have or have not done. He will be there ready to wrap His arms around us if we will invite Him in. His love desires relationship. His love does not force its way upon us. He gives us the choice. He just wants to know us and for us to know Him.

If we choose to reject that relationship, He will let us go

our own way. If we choose to investigate Him, we will begin a lifelong journey of discovery of who God is and of the relationship He desires from us. It will not be a perfect carefree life. However, it will be a life with a companion.

He will walk with us in a spiritual manner that focuses our priorities above the pursuit of personal wealth and pleasure. It is not a life without hardship. It is a place where one can find peace in the midst of trials and hardships.

It is an attitude that rises above our circumstances. It is a relationship not dependent upon our performance. It is a relationship of inward beauty free from the ugliness of surrounding culture.

CHAPTER 9

Sadie

"The love of God is like the Amazon River
flowing down to water one daisy."
- F. B. Meyer

It is early in the morning, the start of a new midsummer pleasant day. The sound of my ringing phone breaks the tranquility of the moment. My friendly greeting to start the conversation is met by a frantic, tired voice. It is Amos. I can hear the distress in his voice.

Amos is a dairyman who recently purchased his farm and dairy cattle. He has a small farm with about 60 cows. He knows his cows. His care for them is exceptional. As with most small dairy farms, he knows his cows as individuals. They are a part of his extended family.

His voice leads directly into a narrative of the events in his life over the past few hours. At 1 a.m., his young son rocks him awake. Their barn is on fire and their cows are in the burning barn. Amos calls the fire company and then along with his son rushes to the barn to rescue his cows. As they enter the burning barn, they encounter billowing, thick smoke. The cows are tethered to their individual stalls. They need to find their way to each cow to unsnap the chain and free them to leave the barn. It is dark. They cannot see and they are chocking on the smoke. For their own safety, they reluctantly abandon the effort. Their barn is ablaze and their family of cows are trapped within.

The firemen soon arrive. They are no stranger to barn fires. These fires happen too commonly in their community. Because hay and straw are so flammable, a fire in a barn catches and erupts quickly. If it is not detected early, the contents including animals are frequently lost. These are true emergencies. Barn fires usually result in the total loss of the building.

The firemen know what to do. They are equipped for the task. Wearing their protective uniforms along with an air supply, they enter the burning barn. They use bolt cutters to sever the chains that tether each cow to her stall. The cows are free to exit the burning inferno. Those that can find their way out of the barn are free to roam around outside wherever they may go.

Amos is concerned about his cows. Some have burns across their back. Most have inhaled a considerable amount of smoke. Many are in distress. He asks me to come to the farm to evaluate his cows and develop a plan to deal with their injuries.

Upon arrival at the farm, I am confronted with the reality of what happened overnight. Friends, family, and neighbors have gathered along with the fire companies to assist in whatever manner they can. They have rounded up the cattle that were in the barn and trucked them to a neighbor's empty barn where they are cared for and fed.

The fire companies are still fighting the fire. The structure of the barn has collapsed inward on itself. Smoke and fire are still billowing among the debris. Some cattle are roaming outside the barn away from the fire. Everyone I meet wears blank concerned expressions on their faces. I roam among the many people seeking the whereabouts of Amos.

Eventually Amos finds me. He is a man of medium stature younger than myself. His face is unusually red. His eyes are bloodshot. He appears exhausted. His clothing is worn and dirty. It is evident that he too has taken in some smoke. He says that he is alright. He informs me that he would like me to travel with him to the neighbor's farm to evaluate his rescued cattle.

We travel to the neighbor's barn to evaluate the cattle. As we travel, I am contemplating how I should go about these evaluations. I need to consider the immediate condition of each cow and I need to consider the long-term prognosis for her health and productivity. I decide that I will triage each cow giving her a score from one to three. A designation of one means the cow is alright and should be kept in the herd. A designation of two means she is distressed but should be given time to heal with the hope that she can remain in the herd. A designation of three means that she needs to be relieved of her misery today and leave the herd. I will examine each cow with an emphasis on the condition of her lungs as well as any external injuries.

We arrive at the neighbor's farm and park outside the barn. The cattle are in a tie-stall barn. There is an ample supply of good feed and water already available to each cow. It is evident that there is a priority to provide care for the cows.

I explain to Amos the procedure that I will use for each cow. He retrieves a tablet and pen to record the evaluations. Amos knows each cow by name. The cows also have individual ear tags with a unique number.

One by one, I examine each cow. From a short distance, I determine her temperament. Most dairy cattle will allow people to approach them gently. They do not like sudden movements and may respond aggressively if threatened. I move closer and take the body temperature. I look over her body for external injuries. I place my stethoscope in my ears and listen to her abdomen and chest. I listen carefully to her lungs and determine her breathing rate and heart rate. After completing my exam, I decide on a triage score, which Amos records for each cow.

I proceed down the long rows of cows. I soon become aware of how well Amos knows his cows. He tells me the name and age of each cow. He tells me about her history in his herd.

He tells me how many calves she has delivered and about other cows related to her that are in the herd. He tells me her importance to his herd production. It seems to me that for every cow, he is begging for a generous score of one or two to keep her in the herd. Many times, there are tears in his eyes and a break in his voice.

As we come to near the end of the first row of cows, Amos steps back, turns away from me, and quietly hesitates from his narrative on each cow. I approach the last cow in this row. He turns back towards me and with more tears in his eyes and a broken voice announces that this is an extra special cow. He has given her a special name. Her name is "Sadie." She is his favorite cow. He tells me much about her. She is the best cow in his herd. It is evident that he is begging for her life to remain with him. As I examine her, I remember that Amos' wife is also named "Sadie." She is indeed very special to him.

As I examine her, I am apprehensive of what I may find. I know his desire. I know that I need to be objective and do what is best for the cow. I listen to her lungs. The breathing is slow and regular. Her lung sounds are normal. I turn back to Amos and with a slight grin, I announce that Sadie… is a one. Amos breaks into a broad smile of relief. Sadie has always been a "one" to Amos.

I complete the task of scoring the cows and most of the cows score a one or two. The firemen have done an exceptional job of retrieving the cows from the burning barn. Just a few cows had been near to where the fire started and are in respiratory distress. They have significant burns. When I announce a score of three, Amos' face turns grim and he quietly moves on to the next cow.

Amos cares for each member of his family of cows. He does not want to lose any of them. His desire is to keep all of them. The reality is that some are saved and some are lost. Nevertheless, life marches onward in spite of his desires. He has to make choices. He can choose to treasure those relationships that are with him. He can choose to release those that are not with him and move on. If he fails to make a choice, he still loses by default.

Our spiritual lives are similar. Whether we acknowledge it or not, there is a spiritual component to our lives. Love and hate exist. Hope and despair exist. Good and evil exist. Mercy and revenge exist. Fear and courage exist. We can explain these away as attitudes and actions derived from emotions or we can acknowledge that our responses arise from the spirit within us. The battle is within us.

We make choices every day as to how we respond to each circumstance. Those choices have a spiritual connection. God will not make the choice for us. He allows us to make the choice. In the same manner, we can choose to know God or to deny Him. His will is that all choose to know Him. Those that make that choice have within them a spirit that chooses love over hate. It chooses good over evil. It chooses mercy over revenge. It chooses courage over fear. It provides hope in place of despair.

If one chooses otherwise, God does not force His way upon them. He waits. Those people go their own way and reap the consequences of their own actions. However, God's love does not end. He will never reject anyone who eventually seeks Him. As illustrated by Amos and Sadie, everyone is special. There is no one that He rejects because they have been separated from Him too long or they feel their life is beyond hope. God does not exist within the constraints of time and space. He is patient. He can wait forever.

From F. B. Meyer, "The love of God is like the Amazon River flowing down to water one daisy." Each person is that one special daisy.

CHAPTER 10

See It to Believe It

"Conversion for me was not a Damascus Road experience.
I slowly moved into an intellectual acceptance
of what my intuition had always known."

- Madeleine L'Engle

I am new to the territory. As a recent graduate from veterinary school and a new addition to the veterinary world, I am under the scrutiny of a microscope. That microscope is the eye of our clientele. They will give you grace for a time. It is alright to say you do not know and I will find the right answer for you. However, do not be wrong.

Gibb is an excellent dairy producer. He takes good care of his cows. When he has a cow with a problem, he calls promptly for service and expects prompt service. Gibb is older than I am. His years of experience have given him confidence in knowing about the problems his cows encounter. He freely expresses his expectations of the vet that is treating his cows. To a young rookie like me, he can be rather intimidating.

Today, Gibb has a cow with a sore foot. Lameness in cattle is a condition that one needs to treat promptly. If left untreated, the cow suffers the misery of the sore foot and becomes unhealthy and unproductive. It is not an emergency but does need treatment before the condition becomes more severe.

I arrive at the farm. As I enter the barn, Gibb's son

meets me and leads me to the patient. He explains that his father is unavailable. However, he expects me to examine and treat the lame cow in his absence. Secretly, I am relieved that I will not need to be under the scrutiny and critical review of Gibb. I can go about my usual procedure for a lame cow without interference.

The cow is in a tie stall. As I approach her, I can see that her left rear foot is swollen above the hoof. At least this rookie will not need to ask which foot is lame. I set my toolbox down a safe distance behind the cow. The stainless steel box contains everything I may need to examine and treat a cow with a sore foot. It contains a variety of hoof knives, files, treatments, bandages, and ropes for restraint.

I open the box and retrieve the rope. I place a loop of the rope below her hock and another loop half hitched above her hock. I attach the free end of the rope to a beam hook attached to a wooden beam above the cow. I elevate and secure the sore foot so that I can safely examine and treat the lameness.

As I clean up the sole of the foot with a hoof knife, I can see that she has an abscess in the sole of her foot. This is quite painful. It is akin to what your thumbnail will feel like if you accidentally strike it with a poorly aimed hammer while attempting to drive a nail into a board. I have done that and borne the pain. To relieve the pain while I open the abscess, I need to anesthetize the foot. I place a tourniquet below her hock and then inject an anesthetic into her vein. This anesthetizes everything below the tourniquet. It relieves the pain and allows me to safely work on the foot without being kicked into oblivion.

I use the hoof knife to pare down to and open the abscess. As I open the abscess there is a burst of fluid from it, releasing the pressure within. I continue to remove hoof material from the sole until there is no undermined cavity remaining on the sole of her foot. When finished, I can see that I have removed a large portion of the sole and exposed a large area of very sensitive flesh underlying the abscess.

To allow the cow to walk comfortably, I cement a block of wood to her good claw so that she can apply weight to the lame foot without walking on the sore claw. I finish the job by applying an antiseptic to the sole and placing a large elastic bandage around the entire foot, effectively covering up everything I have just done. For absent Gibb's benefit, it is out of sight and out of mind. I take a certain amount of pride in my ability to place a bandage on a foot that will stay in place until one forcibly removes it. It will not fall off after I leave the farm.

I release the foot from the restraints and allow the cow to stand on that leg again. I notice that she already feels much better with the ability to stand on that leg without pain. The mission is accomplished without the scrutiny of Gibb. I clean and pack up my tools and without further thought about the foot, proceed with my day.

The next morning starts a new day for this young rookie, who is still learning the tricks of the trade and trying his hardest to gain the confidence of the clients in this profession. Bright and early, the phone rings. It is Gibb. In his rather gruff voice, he exclaims, "Doc, you need to come and put another bandage on that foot you treated yesterday."

I am disappointed in myself. I thought I put a good bandage on that foot that would not fall off on its own accord. My confidence is shaken. I ask, "Did the bandage fall off?"

Gibb is quiet for a moment. Then rather sheepishly, he softly says, "No, I took it off."

Exasperated, I reply, "Why did you do that?"

"I wanted to see what it looked like."

Forcefully, I reply, "Ok, what did it look like?"

With a chuckle, Gibb replied, "It looked like it needed a bandage on it."

We both laugh at his honesty and I agree to come back out and replace the bandage on the foot.

Seeing is believing. Many of us are reluctant to simply accept someone else's view on an issue. We must see something ourselves in order to believe it. It is the difference between being told about an event and experiencing the actual event.

Approaching the possibility of a spiritual reality is like that. Initially, it seems like a long shot. It seems unlikely. It is beyond reason. It seems like something only for the weak, an excuse to escape their troubles. To reach beyond reason for answers is troubling for many. It even seems like an unnecessary crutch for those that are unable to resolve the reality of life in rational terms. Yet, there is an instinctive knowing within us to search for what seems unsearchable.

As one delves into the existence of life on this planet, they discover a detail of complexity that is astounding to a rational mind. Think about the likelihood of life happening as a random event. Start by arranging an assortment of subatomic particles into atoms. Let those atoms form molecules. Those atoms and molecules form a physical substances called matter.

The atoms and molecules, especially carbon, hydrogen, and water, take on a complexity of their own to cross that boundary into living cells. Within the cells are organelles, each with a specific role in the greater function of the cell. The cells take on different expressions of their DNA for the formation of tissues. Each unique tissue contributes to a specific role to form organs in the animal kingdom like a heart, kidney, liver, skin, stomach, intestine, veins and arteries. The organs, each with a specific purpose, arrange into body parts like feet, legs, arms, thorax, abdomen, neck, and a head with facial features that are distinctively unique to each individual to form an organism.

Now enlist neural and hormonal mechanisms to keep the organs functioning at a steady level. Provide for the defense with an immune system that detects the difference between friend and foe. It sustains the friend for survival and resists the foe. Provide for the offense with a reproductive system to continue the line of life with new nearly identical, yet unique individuals to continue the lineage of life. Hide within the organism repair mechanisms that automatically fix broken parts. Then place a brain and spinal cord in charge of the entire fleet to coordinate activities in such a manner that everything works together for the common good.

The same holds true in a much different arrangement of parts for the plant kingdom. There are roots, stems, leaves, flowers, and seeds. The plants capture energy from the sun to provide for food to sustain the animal kingdom. The plant and animal kingdoms have within them a flow of nutrients between species. The nutrients are ultimately recycled back to the earth to be used again in an ongoing cycle of life. One wonders as to what is the impetus that caused all this order to occur. Can it be only by chance alone?

Now, arrange the organisms into species that live together in the same locale each with their own ecological niche. Arrange the species into families and communities with the goal of order for the common good.

At the top of all the life forms, place one greater species with higher intellect to care for and guard the common good. Let it be a species with the ability to discover and understand the intricacies of life and the mechanisms by which that life flourishes on this planet.

Oh, but wait. What will happen if that top of the chain species decides to place their own interests ahead of the common good? The great species begin to quarrel among themselves. They start wars to dominate one another. They take advantage of the less fortunate among them. They abuse the lesser species.

The system originally developed as a self-sustaining system of good that is overseen by the intellect of the great species, is now contaminated with evil. There is a constant conflict between good and evil in their midst. The good and evil amongst them is something that is not composed of the original matter that developed into physical life. It is something different. It is a spiritual reality.

The reality is that physical life on this planet is composed of the substance or matter that forms physical objects. In addition to that, there are nonphysical spiritual forces. There is within that spiritual reality the existence of good and evil. The good we call God. The evil we call sin.

At some point, it becomes more reasonable to believe in a God who engineered this complex system. To not believe in a divine creator is to believe that it all happened spontaneously and without any guidance. It becomes more reasonable to believe in God as the creator than to not believe in Him.

CHAPTER 11

To the Rescue

"Do not fret, for God did not create us to abandon us."
- Michelangelo Buonarotti

The air temperature this afternoon is right on freezing at 32 degrees Fahrenheit and it is snowing. Wet snow covers everything. It is one of those cold, humid, bone chilling, dreary wet days. I have one more call late in the afternoon.

Rob has a cow that has recently delivered a calf. She refuses to eat anything. That is a bad sign. A number of conditions can cause her to lose her appetite. Rob wants her examined to determine the cause of her illness.

I arrive while it is still snowing. I find Rob already busy with the afternoon milking in the milking parlor. He is an experienced dairy producer and watches over his cows carefully. He stops what he is doing to assist me in examining his ill cow. Rob takes me outside the barn to a small shed located just outside the lot where the cows are fed. The lot is full of cows happily eating their feed. The makeshift shed and surrounding area are covered with a fresh blanket of wet snow. There is a single cow in the shed.

Rob tells me the recent history of this cow. Her name is Daisy. She is an older cow. Daisy just delivered her third calf without assistance a week ago. She was healthy until this morning. She has not eaten anything all day today. Daisy is roaming around loose in the makeshift outdoor pen. There is a flimsy single strand of wire across the front of the shed, apparently used as a gate to contain the cow within.

We need to catch Daisy by placing a rope halter on her and tie her to a post on the side of the shed. Rob and I, one on either side of the cow, ease her into a corner. I try to place a loop of the rope halter over her head. I have done this many times. With patience and persistence, a cow will usually give up after a few attempts and allow me to place the halter on her. Just as I nearly ease the halter over Daisy's head, she swings her head away from me, ripping the halter from my hands. She bolts toward the open front of the shed, nearly running over Rob who wisely steps out of her way. Daisy easily breaks through the single strand of wire across the front of the shed. She is now beyond our control and free to roam wherever her feet may take her. We both leave the shed seeking to corral her back into the shed.

Daisy stops for a moment to plan her next move. Then she turns and flees towards the safety of her herd in the lot nearby. Just as she runs beside the shed, Daisy drops out of sight. She vanishes into an apparent hole in the snow-covered landscape. Rob and I run to find her. We find ourselves peering down into a pit filled with liquid cow waste. The pit had a flimsy cover over it that was hidden by the snow. Daisy stepped on the cover and fell into the pit. As we look down, we can see Daisy a few feet below us swimming in the liquid manure.

This is a bad situation. We have a 1,500-pound cow swimming in cold liquid waste in a pit that, for our own safety, we should not enter. We need to rescue Daisy. She is much too heavy for a man to lift out of the pit. It is cold wet and snowy. Daisy will soon be tired and get hypothermia swimming in the cold liquid waste.

It occurs to me that we often use a device called a hip lift to elevate cows that are unable to stand. This device is clamped over a cow's hipbones. It can be attached to anything that will lift a 1,500-pound cow. I discuss this idea with Rob. We develop a quick plan. I will make a quick trip back to our nearby veterinary office to retrieve a hip lift. Rob will drive a tractor up to the pit with the loader on the front of the tractor directly over Daisy. He volunteers to descend into the pit to place the hip lift on Daisy. This is dangerous. There are often dangerous gasses in the pit. We will place a rope around Rob to pull him to safety if he needs a quick escape. Once the hip lift is secured to Daisy, we will use the lift on the front of the tractor to elevate Daisy out of the pit.

We have a plan. Rob's two sons come to help us. I fetch the hip lift. Rob throws a sheet of plywood down into the pit next to Daisy to give him some flotation while placing the hip lift. Daisy is still swimming. Rob, with safety rope attached, lowers himself into the pit. He kneels on the plywood. His weight causes the plywood to sink a few inches but Rob persists. He successfully places the hip lift on swimming Daisy and attaches a chain to the lift.

We pull Rob back up out of the pit. He is covered with the liquid waste. We attach the chain to the lift on the tractor. Rob slowly engages the lift to elevate Daisy out of the pit. She is cold, wet and miserable. We place Daisy in a warm pen in the barn, clean the waste off of her, and place a blanket on her. I do an examination of her. I decide that it is best to allow her to recover from her ordeal without further intervention today.

I return to Rob's farm the next day. After I examine her, I determine that she needs surgery to correct a twist of her fourth stomach. The procedure is routine. I do them quite often. Daisy recovers from her swimming ordeal. She returns to the herd.

While the analogy is messy and crude, it illustrates how God has not given up on people. In spite of our rejection of God, He wants us back. His love for every human is not conditional. He wants to rescue humans from their descent into the messy waste pit they have made of their lives because of their own choice to abandon their relationship with God.

He chose to become one of us in the life of Jesus Christ. He chose to elevate humanity back into relationship with Him by becoming one of them. To believe that the life and teachings of Jesus are real requires one to believe that there is a reality beyond the natural world, a spiritual reality unseen by our eyes, yet perceived in our spirit. It is a step of faith.

One crosses that barrier in many ways. For some it is a simple willingness to take that step to see what happens to their life. For others it is a drawn-out process of searching for truth. A life-altering calamity may force one to search for answers to questions that plague them. A disgust for failure to achieve happiness through the pursuit of pleasure and wealth may cause one to search for purpose beyond their own natural desires and abilities. It may be a desire to find an absolute truth aside from popular culture.

Anything that sets the search in motion can lead to a fascination of ancient scriptures and archaeological findings. There are many events prophesied hundreds of years before they occurred with amazing accuracy. I have a tendency to be skeptical. My first inclination is to dismiss the fulfillment of these prophesies as mere coincidence. However, at some point, one concludes that it is more rational to believe in their credibility than to dismiss them as coincidence.

The Old Testament books of Hosea and Isaiah were written in the 700s BC. They contain many prophesies that were fulfilled starting about 100 years later and continue to be fulfilled even to the current day.

In the 700s BC the Northern Kingdom of 10 tribes of Israel was overthrown by the Assyrians and led into captivity. They were assimilated into other cultures and lost their identity. The Southern Kingdom of Judah remained. Prophesied in Hosea 1:6, 7.

About 600 BC the remaining tribe of Judah was overcome by the Babylonians and exiled from their land. After 70 years of captivity, the Jews were allowed to return to Jerusalem in 537 BC as prophesied 70 years earlier by both Isaiah and Jeremiah. The return led by Ezra was a revival of the Jewish people and resulted in rebuilding the Temple.

The Jews inhabited the land until 70 AD when the Romans overthrew Jerusalem. A small contingent remained until they were removed in 130 AD.

The land of Israel became a dried-up wasteland for the next 1,800 years. In 1867, Mark Twain visited the area and described what he saw. "A desolation is here that not even imagination can grace with the pomp of life and action. We never saw a human being on the whole route. There was hardly a tree or shrub anywhere." From *The Innocents Abroad* London 1881.

Isaiah 11:11 states that Israel will return a second time. That return began to happen in the late 1800s and peaked after the Soviet Union fell in 1989. From 1989 until 1995, 1.2 million Jews immigrated to Israel from Russia.

From Isaiah 35:1-2: "The wilderness and the dry land shall be glad; The desert shall rejoice and blossom on the growth of Israel." For this prophesy to be fulfilled it will take a lot of water.

Israel's source of fresh water is the Sea of Galilee. By the 1980s the fresh water supply was being depleted faster than it was replenished. Since that time, Israel has developed wastewater reclamation technologies, drip line irrigation, and saltwater desalination plants to bolster their water supply. By 2023 they are producing 20% more water than they are consuming.

In March of 2024 I had the opportunity to visit the Negev Desert in southern Israel for a service project. I worked in the greenhouses. The desert is blooming abundantly. Isaiah's prophesy is being fulfilled 2,600 years later. It is an exciting time to see that come about.

God created this planet and the life forms that exist on it.

It may have been instant in six simple days. It may have been in six extended eras of evolving time. He placed humanity as the highest intelligent species on this planet. His desire was for humanity to live their lives in relationship with God, inspired and in awe of the beauty of His creation. He gave humanity the freedom to choose to be in that relationship or to reject Him. Humanity chose to go their own way and reject God. However, they still had a spirit within them. They searched for their own gods in many ways. They still are doing that. God wants them back. He came as one of us to provide a way back into relationship with Him. God created people in His own image. He created people to have a spirit within them. People are the most important thing to Him. That is love.

CHAPTER 12

A Two Beer Calving

"The two most important days in our life
are the day we are born...
and the day we find out why."

- Mark Twain

Emergency calls are a necessity in the routine of a full-service veterinarian. Where there is life, there will be situations that require immediate intervention. While these calls can come at some of the most inconvenient times, they do take precedence over whatever else one may be doing.

It is Friday. This is my weekend to be on call for emergencies. I will be on call from Friday morning until Monday morning. Our answering service sends us calls with a text message. I have programmed my cell phone with a unique notification alert specifically for text messages from our answering service. That alert is a rendition of "Who Let the Dogs Out?"

As my phone chirps up with "Who Let the Dogs Out?," I know I have a Friday evening call to start the weekend. I open my text application to read a message indicating that Bud has a cow in labor that is not progressing with a normal delivery of the calf. There is no need to return his phone call. Just come to the farm ASAP.

As I travel the short distance to Bud's farm, I consider the likely calving scenarios that I may be about to encounter. Every calving is an adventure. One never know what lies ahead until arrival at the farm and examination of the cow.

Upon examination of cow number 747, I determine that she has a uterine torsion. She is a huge cow. I am about to engage in another calving adventure.

A uterine torsion occurs when the calf and the womb flip inside the cow and create a functional obstruction to the delivery. It is impossible to deliver the calf because the birth canal is narrowed by the torsion. Correction of the torsion requires flipping the entire mass of calf and womb back into a normal position.

A common way to do this is to lie the cow down and roll her over her back while securing the womb with a plank laid across her lower abdomen. We call this procedure: "Planking the Cow." This requires at least three people and a lot of muscle to accomplish the task. One person to roll the front of the cow, another on the back of the cow, and the third person to stand on the plank laid across the abdomen. As the cow is rolled over her back, the womb is held steady in place. Essentially one holds the womb in place with the plank and turns the cow.

An alternative procedure is to secure the calf with a rod and calving chains on the feet of the calf and turn the calf and womb inside the cow. This requires internal access to the calf. If the cervix is too narrow, this is not possible.

Bud, his brother, and his nephew are all present as I inform them of the diagnosis. Number 747 is a very large 1,800-pound cow. The three of them are familiar with uterine torsions. They know the possible procedures and the effort required to "plank" a large cow.

It's Friday evening after a long workweek. They jokingly tease that they are not up to the exertion of rolling an 1,800-pound cow. They prefer the rod approach.

To that end, they challenge me with a bargain. "If you can get the torsion untwisted without the need to roll the cow, we will give you one beer. To sweeten the challenge, if you deliver a live calf we will give you a second beer. There is a case of beer in the office. We have the goods to back up the deal."

I am challenged to a "Two Beer Calving." With a mischievous grin, I jokingly accept the deal.

From my examination of the cow, I already know that I have access to the calf to apply the calving chains on the feet. I should be able to correct the torsion without the need to roll the cow. That will be worth one beer.

I proceed to secure the calf with obstetrical chains and attach the chains to the rod. I grab the rod and start to rock the mass of calf and womb back and forth until I complete the flip to correct the torsion. I reexamine the cow and determine that the procedure is successful. Great, one beer earned.

Now it is just a matter of slowly assisting the cow as she finishes dilating and delivering the calf. She has been in labor for an extended time. The calf may be deceased. I do not feel any movement of the calf during the delivery. This is not unusual, but without movement, it may mean that it is too late to deliver a live calf.

I deliver the calf. It does not breathe immediately. I touch the cornea of one eye. The calf blinks. I tickle the nose. The calf shakes its head and takes a deep breath. After a slight pause, I tickle its nose again and rub its chest. It takes another breath and then begins to breathe in a regular pattern. The calf is alive. It is a successful "Two Beer Calving." True to their promise, Bud and company cheerfully deliver on their end of the bargain.

We like to make deals to get what we desire. We do it when we make a purchase. We do it with friends and family. If you do something for me, I will return the favor to you. Without being aware of it, we often approach God in the same way. If I am good today, show me your favor. If I am good and put something in the offering at church, will You show me your favor by getting me a better job? We do it in our prayers. I was good today. I went to church instead of the golf course. Now will You fix my marriage?

The "Kingdom of Self" initiates many of the motivations of mankind. Even our charitable activities may be driven through a desire for recognition and approval from other people. It makes us feel we are good. The focus is on what we receive through our words and actions.

It is easy to approach God the same way. There are times that we fail to fulfill our end of our perceived bargain with God. It will happen, and when it does, we expect God to withdraw His approval from us.

That is not the way God works. The "Kingdom of God" is not like that. His kingdom is not of this natural world. To find it, we must reach beyond the natural world to discover a spiritual reality seen only by the spirit within us. His favor, His love, His guidance, His protection, and His healing power are not dependent on what we do. The very act of trying to strike up a deal with God is offensive to who He is and the relationship He desires to have with those who choose to follow Him.

God's favor is not conditional. It is free because of His love for people. It is the grace of God. We cannot buy it. We cannot earn it. We cannot strike a deal to get it. We cannot impose our own will and desires on God. We cannot tell Him what His will for our circumstance should be. We can only come to Him with a humble request for His will in our circumstance. He does not impose His will. He waits for people to choose to come to Him. When we give up our will and accept His will, we are freed from the condemnation of failure.

Who is this God? Who is this Jesus? Consider this description from a sermon by S. M. Lockridge entitled "He's My King." It is often referred to as "The Greatest Sermon Ever Preached." What follows is his description of God.

"He's enduringly strong, He's entirely sincere, He's eternally steadfast. He's immortally graceful. He's imperially powerful. He's impartially merciful. He's God's Son. He's a sinner's savior. He's the centerpiece of civilization. He stands alone in Himself. He's unparalleled. He's unprecedented. He's supreme. He's preeminent. He's the loftiest idea in literature. He's the highest idea in philosophy. He's the fundamental truth in theology. He's the miracle of the age. He's the only one able to supply all of our needs simultaneously. He supplies strength for the weak. He's available for the tempted and the tried. He sympathizes and He saves. He guards and He guides. He heals the sick, He cleans the lepers. He forgives sinners, He discharges debtors, He delivers captives, He defends the feeble, He blesses the young, He serves the unfortunate, He regards the aged, He rewards the diligent, He beautifies the meek. Do you know Him?

"Well, my king is the king of knowledge, He's the wellspring of wisdom, He's the doorway of deliverance, He's the pathway of peace, He's the roadway of righteousness, He's the highway of holiness, He's the gateway of glory, He's the master of the mighty, He's the captain of the conquerors, He's the head of the heroes, He's the leader of the legislators, He's the overseer of the overcomers, He's the governor of governors, He's the prince of princes, He's the king of Kings and the Lord of Lords.

"His life is matchless. His goodness is limitless. His mercy is everlasting. His love never changes. His word is enough. His grace is sufficient. His reign is righteous. His yoke is easy and His burden is light. Well. I wish I could describe Him to you. But He's indescribable. Yes. He's incomprehensible. He's invincible, He's irresistible. I'm trying to tell you, the Heavens cannot contain Him, let alone a man explain Him. You can't get Him out of your mind. You can't get Him off of your hands. You can't outlive Him, and you can't live without Him. Well. The Pharisees couldn't stand Him, but they found out they couldn't stop Him. Pilate couldn't find any fault in Him. Herod couldn't kill Him. Death couldn't handle Him and the grave couldn't hold Him. That's my king!

"He always has been, and He always will be. I'm talking about He [who] had no predecessor and He [who] has no successor. There was nobody before Him and there will be nobody after Him. You can't impeach Him, and He's not going to resign. We try to get prestige and honor and glory to ourselves, but the glory is all His. Thine is the kingdom and the power and the glory forever, and ever, and ever, and ever. How long is that? And ever, and ever, and ever, and ever, and when you get through with all of the forevers, then 'Amen'.

"Oh I wish I could describe him to you."

- Dr. Shadrach Meshach (S. M.) Lockridge (March 7, 1913–April 4, 2000)

CHAPTER 13

Fitting In

"Nobody goes there anymore because it's too crowded."
- Yogi Berra

I am given another opportunity to travel to a central Asian country to serve as a resource to their dairy industry. It is an honor to be asked to serve in this manner. The country is Turkmenistan. It is essentially a dry barren desert that is sandwiched between Afghanistan, Iran, Uzbekistan, and the Caspian Sea.

The country of Turkmenistan was a member of the former Soviet Union. It is sparsely populated with about six million people. The Black Sand Desert covers most of the country's land-locked area. It has a totalitarian government. It has been criticized for its poor record on human rights.

I fly a circuitous route to the capitol city of Turkmenistan, Ashgabat. I fly first to Germany, then to Turkey, and after a long layover in Istanbul, I arrive at my destination.

Going through customs is a bit nerve-wracking for me because you never know what to expect. My luggage consists of clothing, a computer, and some small gifts to give to my hosts and the farms I will visit.

In customs, I am asked to step to the side for a detailed inspection. Several agents open all my luggage and root through everything. None of them speaks English. They find a small cardboard box. They motion for me to open it. It contains chocolate candy from Hershey, PA, USA. I thought that would be a special treat for those I meet. I open the box and ask them to help themselves. They all break into smiles and decline the offer.

That was the end of the inspection and they motion for me to continue into their country. I am met by a driver to take me to my destination.

Ashgabat is ornate. There are pristine marble buildings and golden domes along wide boulevards and manicured gardens. I frequently see women in burkas that are tasked with cleaning the streets. Their only tool is a small broom. There is no litter, no graffiti, and no crime. I see police on almost every street corner.

There are fountains spouting water into the dry air everywhere. It seems like a celebration of water in the desert. Two canals of water, one in the north, and another in the south supply water to the country. It is very hot, but it is a dry heat.

I meet my contact, Joe, who takes me to lunch at a local sandwich shop. I am exhausted from jet lag but appreciative of the company of an English-speaking person. It gets very lonely when one is not able to communicate in the company of people that speak a different language. I want to fit in with the group, but I am left alone because of the language barrier.

I know Joe from a previous trip to Kazakhstan. He is the one that recruited me for this opportunity. Joe has a heart for assisting agriculture in developing countries. Joe tells me that this trip is going to be different. In Kazakhstan, we assisted large government dairy farms. This time we are going out into the communities to serve the little people.

I sense a bit of resentment in Joe for overbearing governments. He wants to help the community people. Extended families live in small compounds consisting of a house and several outbuildings to house their livestock. Many have a couple of cows, camels, goats, and sheep. Each family compound is enclosed in a tall wooden fence. There is a locked gate for entry from the village road. Every morning the village children gather the cows from several compounds and shepherd them to pastures outside the village to graze for the day.

My mission with Joe is to assist a new cheese making enterprise to acquire more quality milk to meet the demand for cheese. This small business has been very successful selling cheese. They acquire milk from the small family compounds. They have asked for more milk to meet the growing demand for cheese.

The families have agreed to supply more milk, by adding water to the existing supply. Obviously, that is not in the interests of the cheese business. My task is to show these small farms how to produce more quality milk from their cows, without adding water to the milk they ship to the cheese plant. It is a nutritional problem. I need to show them how to feed their cows a better diet to produce more milk.

The plan is to work with local villagers to set up demonstration trials in three areas of the country. We hope to motivate the villagers to produce more milk of a good quality suitable for making cheese. The three areas are long distances apart. One is in the North, near Uzbekistan. Another is in the South near Iran. The third is in the East near Afghanistan.

Transportation to these three areas is by air. As we fly to each area, I see endless stretches of nothing by dry desert sand. There are no roads. The areas we travel to are located near the two canals that carry water from mountains located east of the country.

Each farm we visit is welcoming. I tour the farm, gather information, and return the next day with a plan for the feeding trial. The objective is to improve the milk production of their cows.

The culmination of each visit is a meal with the host. We recline on the floor around a large Persian carpet covered with dishes of vegetables, mutton, and beef. The guest offers a toast to the host and the meal begins. Conversation is abundant. Much of it is in Russian. The Russian language is of a Slavic origin. It is not of a Latin origin. It is difficult for me to understand the conversations. Consequently, I remain quiet until spoken to in the English language. The causal give and take of family conversation does not include me.

On one such occasion, everyone is given a bowl of milk. The host explains to me that it is fermented camel milk. It is a health food. He confidently explains that it is "good for you." Everyone around the table gleefully drinks from their bowl of fermented camel's milk.

I hesitate. The better sense of my inner voice tells me to avoid it. Milk is a rich media for growing bacteria and pathogens. Everyone is looking at me. Again, I am encouraged to consume their health food. It is good for you. I hesitate, but the adventurous spirit in me concedes that I probably will never again have such an opportunity to consume fermented camel's milk. I smile and gleefully drink the milk.

The next day I regret it. I come down with the worst case of traveler's diarrhea I have ever had. I am miserable. We visit other families and I frequent their bathrooms. Fortunately, I have some medicine that the USA travel clinic gave me for just this purpose. After a few days, I am fully recovered.

I had succumbed to peer pressure. I wanted to fit in. I did not want to disappoint my hosts. I wanted to be part of the crowd.

People are social beings. We like to be part of the group. Taking a stand apart from the popular culture is difficult. We have an inner voice to guide us if we choose to listen to that inner voice. If we cultivate that voice, it will be for our benefit. If we constantly suppress that voice, it will eventually disappear. Life is a continuum of choices. The choices we make lead our lives in specific directions. It can be for our betterment or it can be to our eventual demise.

The irony of Yogi Bera's pronouncement is that the crowd is there and that is the reason he states that nobody goes there. Many people choose to follow the popular crowd. The individual decides to avoid the crowd. Something within them kept them from following the crowd. Popular culture tells us that God is nothing more than an ancient tradition, fantasized by generations of uninformed civilizations. It is easy to accept the path of that crowd. It takes effort to delve deep into the issue and make our own decision, unbiased by popular culture.

CHAPTER 14

Oblivious

"I believe in Christianity as I believe that the sun has risen:
not only because I see it,
but because by it I see everything else."

- C. S. Lewis

(From *Is Theology Poetry?*, 1945)

I need at least five hours of uninterrupted sleep to be able to fully function in my duties the next day. I prefer more than that, but I can function one day on that amount of sleep. If I retire at 10 p.m., that means I need until at least 3 a.m. for the five hours.

It is 1 a.m. My work phone blasts through the quietness with its disturbing notification rendition of "Who Let the Dogs Out?" In my slumber, I stumble to consciousness to find the phone and answer with a bleary "Hello."

The first words in my ear are: "Hey Doc, I need you to come to my farm ASAP for a cow trying to deliver a calf. She has been working on it since yesterday afternoon and nothing has happened."

As I gain consciousness and civility, I get his name and location and agree to come to the farm now. I stumble through the dark to find clothing appropriate for a dark, cold, wet night. I try to be quiet so as not to disturb Joyce. Eventually I am prepared for the trip. As I travel to the farm, I make a concerted effort to adjust my attitude and demeanor to something more appropriate.

Wally is an older dairyman. His farm has been in the family for generations and nothing has changed for generations. The buildings are from a former era. I enter the barn through a creaky door that is off of one hinge. The bottom of the door drags on the ground with a screech as I open it. I am wide awake now. I am ready to allow myself to slip into an automatic mode, brought on by years of experience with calvings.

Wally's face shows the wrinkles of years of hard labor in the sun. He cares for his cows and his expression of concern ignites a sense of compassion for him within me. Wally hurries me along to a pen in the back of his barn. There is a single incandescent light bulb in the far corner of the pen. It is dark. Before me is a high wooden obstruction. It is taller than I am. It is a hayrack. There is a trough below it where grain is fed to the cow.

Wally instructs me that the cow is in a pen on the other side of the hayrack and that the entrance to the pen is obstructed. I will need to climb over the hayrack to gain entrance into the pen. It is the only way into the pen. Wally's concern urges me on. I grab the top of the hayrack above my head and launch myself onto the top of the hayrack.

As I gaze down into the dark pen from my perch, I can dimly see a cow gazing up at my intrusion. She stands directly in front of me. As my eyes adjust to the poor lighting, I notice some movement beside her. It is a wet newborn calf shaking its head as it adjusts to the realities of life outside the womb. The cow looks good and the calf has already arrived. I am done with this emergency. A sense of relief comes over me as I know that I can return home to my slumber without getting wet and dirty from a prolonged midnight calving. My mood is much brighter.

I cheerfully announce to Wally that the cow has already

delivered a healthy calf. We can both return to our restful sleep knowing that all is well. A slight grin of relief washes over the concern on his face. As I drop down from my perch, Wally hesitates and then responds.

"What if she has twins? Could you check for another calf?"

I am in automatic mode. I just want to return to my car and drive home. It is the eerie dark of early morning. Reluctantly and hypocritically, I cheerfully concede to his request.

I return to the hayrack. I pull myself back up to perch on top of the rack. I am of a one-track mind. I will make a quick exam for another calf and I am done. I am oblivious to everything else.

The cow is directly facing me. She is glaring at me. I need to drop down into the pen to examine her for a second calf. I want to get this over with. My slumber beckons me back to my home. Most dairy cows are accustomed to being with people and tolerate the presence of a person nearby.

I abandon my perch on top of the hayrack and drop to one side of the cow, careful to not land directly in front of her. As my feet touch the ground, she turns toward me and with head lowered, charges directly at me. Instinctively, I move to her side and behind her. She does not retreat but keeps up her frontal attack. She tries to obtain a head-on attack as I keep moving to her side and behind her. Round and round we go. She is not giving up. This is one mad momma bear. I am in a confined space with no easy way out.

For my own safety, I need to find a way out of here. The gate to the pen is obstructed and I cannot exit that way. The only way out is the way I came in, over the top of the hayrack. She outweighs me ten to one. The only option is escape. As I make a pass by the high hayrack and bolstered by an adrenalin surge, I launch myself upwards to grab the top of the rack. As I pull myself upward to the safety of my perch, I expect to feel her head smash into my legs, shattering one or both knees. To my relief, the cow hesitates as I pull myself up out of danger. That was a close call.

I am breathing heavily. My adrenalin-fueled "flight or fight" response is entirely driven by flight. I look down into the dark pen. The cow is glaring at me, still directly facing me. I can read her body language. "Do not even think about coming back down here."

Wally has been watching this with amusement. It will make a great story to tell his friends and neighbors about the time his cow took on the vet, and won.

I respond wide-eyed and annoyed, "Wally, I am done with this. I am not checking her for twins."

Wally chuckles and thanks me as I leave the barn.

There is a rule about calvings. After delivering a calf, always check for another calf. On my drive home, I feel remorse on not having followed through on that rule. In retrospect, I could have persisted to safely move the cow to another location, secure her in such a way that she cannot attack, and complete the examination. I dismiss the thought. Although twins are quite common, the odds are that she did not have twins.

As I go about my work the next day, the question lingers in my mind. I need to be reassured that the cow is alright. After my morning calls, I return to Wally's farm. I enter the barn and walk to the back pen. As I climb to my perch on top of the hayrack, I see momma cow bright and alert basking in the sunlight. She has two lively calves contently nursing on her, one on each side. She did have twins. Thankfully, she was able to deliver both of them without assistance.

The daily grind is a big part of our lives. We get in a rut of doing the same thing repeatedly each day. Our reactions become automatic with little thought of change.

I was mentally shortsighted about the possible danger of dropping into Wally's pen. I plowed ahead with my own agenda without thought. I just wanted to get done. I failed to adequately evaluate a new circumstance. I stuck with what I have always done. I nearly paid a nasty price for my inattention to change my ways.

Our thoughts and beliefs are like that also. In our youth, we develop a core value system of beliefs. This is who I am. This is what I have always done. This is what I believe. It will not change. If a challenge arises that should cause me to reconsider what I have always believed, I will not change my stance on my beliefs. Our culture considers that stance a strength of character. It is humbling to do otherwise.

Many people are firmly entrenched on both, or many, sides of the Christian debate. It is beyond reason to believe that there is a spiritual reality. It is beyond reason to believe there is a God who became a man. It is beyond reason to believe that God existed in the person of Jesus. It is beyond reason to believe that Jesus performed miracles that defied the laws of physics. It is beyond reason to believe that after Jesus was killed in a gruesome manner, He left the grave and regained life. It is beyond reason to believe there is a God who sent Him to us specifically to restore a spiritual relationship with humanity. It is beyond reason to believe that a man with no formal education could impact the history of the entire world for over 2,000 years. However, Jesus did change the course of human history for over 2,000 tears.

With such an impact on world history, it implores every human to examine the archeological evidence, secular historical evidence, and the biblical prophecy concerning the life of Jesus along the timeline of history. The consequences of living a life in a daily monotonous grind without engaging the question of Jesus are enormous.

At some point along that journey, it becomes more rational to believe, than to not believe. For some it requires a longstanding and painstaking effort to discover truth. For others, it is a simple step of faith. No one will get it perfectly right.

We need only to agree that we are all in a lifelong journey to discover absolute truth and that there will be differences of opinion among us. Let us not focus on the differences and let them discourage and divide us.

There should not be conflict between scientific truth and biblical truth. Truth is true regardless of how the discovery comes about. The conflict comes when conjecture and opinion present themselves as absolute truth. If God created it all, then somehow, scientific and biblical truth must co-exist as one truth. For now, we see in part. Someday we will see the whole.

The central question that unites Christians is a belief in God who came as a man among us in order to make us aware of a spiritual reality and bring us back into relationship with Him. That is the thumbs up or down question. If I say that I do believe in Jesus, but I am wrong, then when breath passes from me, I will no longer exist and awareness of reality will cease. That will be the end and I will not be aware of anything else. Dust to dust with a nonspiritual life in between the beginning and the end.

If I am right about Jesus, then when the breath passes from me, I am freed from the constraints of time and space. My spirit enters a new reality that is far beyond the beauty of this earth. It is beyond imagination. It is not bound by the limits of time. It is eternal, glorious, and wonderful, without fear, without heartache, without disease, without evil, and more glorious than we can now imagine.

If there is a spiritual reality and I make the wrong decision by denying Jesus, that will send me into a dark spirituality filled with all the bad things. At some point, it becomes more rational to believe, than to not believe. To be oblivious to the issue is to lose the rewards. The consequences are eternal.

The human condition that obstructs one from taking that step of faith is pride. To declare that our faith is in something other than our own reason and abilities is seen by some as a weakness. Society encourages individuals to develop confidence in themselves. To proclaim a belief in something we do not fully understand is admitting that we draw strength from something beyond ourselves.

To the contrary, there is a strength in admitting that one has not yet undertaken the effort to examine the prophetic and historical evidence. There is strength in departing from the daily grind to come to a decision that may change your belief system forever. The unforeseen aspect of such an endeavor is that as one begins that process, God will meet you. He will show Himself to you personally in ways you would never suspect. Within you, a confidence and peace overtake the daily grind. That transformation will only occur once the individual decides to begin the process.

As C. S. Lewis said, "I believe in Christianity as I believe that the sun has risen: not only because I see it, but because by it I see everything else."

Once one takes that step, our eyes open to a whole new perspective on life. We see things differently. We see them from a more purposeful and eternal perspective. We still struggle with the same failures, disappointments, heartaches, diseases, and shortcomings that everyone else does. However, our perspective is different in a way that those things do not utterly destroy us.

The decision to believe or not to believe in Christ is critical. If I choose to not believe and I am wrong, I am doomed to an afterlife that has been described as a pit of eternal fire. It is hell.

If I choose to believe and I am wrong, then when life is over, my consciousness will cease and I will never know the difference.

If I choose to believe in Christ and I am right, the reward is an afterlife so glorious and indescribable that I do not want to take the chance of missing it.

CHAPTER 15

Fear and Courage

"Courage is not simply one of the virtues,
but the form of every virtue at the testing point."

\- C. S. Lewis

Every day I work with cattle. They are what I do. Occasionally a call comes in to work on a different species. It is exciting to have such an opportunity. It presents a new challenge to spice up an otherwise routine day.

Most people like animals. A business that allows people to interact with animals has a competitive edge over one without that draw. This is the case for Mikey's food stand. Mikey is a nice middle-aged fellow with a food stand surrounded by an assortment of animals in wide-open areas for people to see. There are geese, ducks, sheep, goats, and deer.

The main attraction is a large black bear named Brutus, residing in a specially-built residence. Brutus is a longtime resident of Mikey's food court. Brutus is often the subject of families taking selfies of themselves with Brutus on the inside of the fence and the family safely on the outside.

Mikey's call was a special request. He needs to make some repairs to Brutus' residence. He called to ask if we could tranquilize Brutus to allow the repairs to be completed while Brutus slept. This is a new and exciting challenge. We have never tended to a bear.

Three veterinarians, Bridget, Mary, and myself, from our large animal veterinary clinic travel to Mikey's business. Upon arrival, we notice the usual gathering of fascinated customers surrounding Brutus. Also present is a work crew waiting to make repairs to an area where the floor is cracked.

The plan is simple. Administer a tranquilizer to Brutus. Allow him to fall asleep and then move him safely to a corner of the pen to allow repairs. Bridget will load a dart with a tranquilizer and use a dart gun to administer the dart from a safe distance.

The crew that is to fix the flooring in the pen is impatiently waiting for Brutus' slumber. They are anxious to get to work. Mikey gives us permission to proceed with our part of the task. There is a growing audience of Mikey's customers.

Brutus is active. He walks about putting on a show for the unusually large crowd gathered to watch the event. The dart is loaded with tranquilizer and placed properly into the dart gun. Ready, aim, and fire. The dart hits the bear and bounces off his tough hide. He does not receive the proper dose.

We reload and try again with the same result. We are frustrated at our inability to administer the tranquilizer to Brutus from a safe distance. We repeat the procedure a few more times with the same result. It seems that the dart gun is not designed with enough power for Brutus. The audience is still growing and becoming more amused at our predicament. It is evident that we are not able to dart Brutus.

The three frustrated veterinarians retreat to discuss the situation. Our plan has failed. The sensible decision is to call it an unsuccessful mission, acquire a more powerful dart gun, and return another day.

Mikey and the work crew are still waiting for us to get Brutus out of their way. The only other option is to take a syringe loaded with a hefty dose of tranquilizer and go directly into the pen with the bear to deliver the shot. No one wants to go into the pen with the bear. The flooring crew is anxious to start repairs. We are anxious to leave our embarrassment behind us.

After some thought about how to approach Brutus, I reluctantly decide to cautiously go into the pen. I will observe Brutus' reaction to my intrusion. If appropriate, I will quietly approach him, administer the shot while he is distracted from outside the pen, and then exit before he reacts aggressively.

I have never done anything like this. My emotions are a combination of intrigue and substantial fear. Brutus is in a corner facing away from the entrance door.

I load a syringe with the tranquilizer. I quietly open the door. Brutus is distracted by all the activity away from me. I hesitate for a moment, watching his reaction. He seems oblivious to my presence in the pen.

It is time to make my move. Mary throws a blanket over the fence. As the blanket descends on Brutus' head, I quickly move to Brutus, remove the needle cap, and thrust the needle into Brutus' backside. I push the plunger on the syringe to deliver the tranquilizer.

I do not know what to expect as a bear has never attacked me. Fearing the worst reaction from Brutus, I turn and run for my life fearing the bear attack soon to inevitably follow. Without looking back, I race through the door and slam it closed behind me. Only then, from safely outside, do I turn and look back over my shoulder.

Brutus is still in the corner. He shakes the blanket off his body and turns to look at me, seemingly puzzled at what just happened. He rises to stroll around the pen. Slowly he begins to feel the effect of the tranquilizer. He lies down and quietly loses awareness of everything around him.

The three of us go into the pen to move him safely away from the area in need of repairs. Finally, the work crew is able to enter the pen to complete their repairs. Brutus sleeps for a long time. Eventually he will wake up to resume his entertainment of customers.

Fear of bodily harm and the courage to resist that fear are a battle that occurs within our minds. It is a battle within our spirit. These inward battles precede many of our responses to the challenges of daily living.

There is a story in the Bible that exemplifies this inward battle. It is recorded in the Gospel of Mathew 16:16-23. Jesus asks the disciples who they think He is. Peter responds that Jesus is the Messiah, the Son of the living God. Jesus is delighted in Peter's answer and responds that Peter is not given that insight by his own mind. Rather God reveals it to him.

Jesus then tells Peter about His forthcoming betrayal and crucifixion. Peter responds with a very human declaration that he will stand in Jesus' defense and never let that happen. Jesus responds forcefully with "Get thee behind me, Satan."

Jesus is not calling Peter Satan. He is speaking directly to the source of Peter's response. In one moment, Peter's thoughts switch from hearing God in his mind to hearing Satan in his mind. Peter verbalized the battles in his mind.

In Ephesians 6:12, Paul refers to these battles within our spirit. "For our battle is not against flesh and blood, but against the rulers, against the authorities, against the powers of this dark world and against the spiritual forces of evil in the heavenly realms."

In the experience with Brutus the bear, I had to choose between the voice of fear and the voice of courage in my mind. The actions were merely the result of that choice. Whether we are aware of it or not, the real battle starts in our minds before we engage the natural world around us. It is evidence of the spiritual reality. If we accept that there is a spiritual reality, then we must come to a decision concerning what we will choose to believe about the reality of God and about the inward battles that we encounter.

The battle is often a conflict between truths and lies. The forces of evil bombard our minds with lies. They tell us there is no God. If there is a God, you are too insignificant for Him to care about you. You have not earned His favor. Everyone hates you. They laugh at you behind your back. These are the tools of Satan to destroy you. They are based upon thoughts about ourselves and our worth. They substitute self-awareness for God awareness.

If we choose to look to God for our worth, it frees us from the noose of seeking worth from our peers. Instead, the Holy Spirit within us prompts us to truths about God, specifically His love for all people as individuals regardless of their circumstances. Our value depends upon a love that will not be withdrawn because of performance.

We are brought to a place of remorse for our failures to truly follow the Holy Spirit's promptings. That is called repentance. What follows is a desire to be more aware of and follow God's leading in our lives. We do not always get it right. Therefore, we come back to repentance.

There is a spiritual power struggle within our minds between God and Satan. It implores us to engage those battles with the weapons God provides. Jesus is the source of God-given power to overcome the forces of evil. There are times when one must directly refute the lies by citing the truths of Jesus' life. He is God come to people as a person. He lived among us. He taught us about God. He gave His physical life through rejection and torture to die a gruesome physical death to pay the price for all of mankind's sin. Then He defeated the power of death through His resurrection.

We call upon that power to resist the lies that attempt to destroy us. We do that by reminding spiritual forces of darkness that we align with Jesus. On that authority, we refuse to believe the lies. We resist them by the authority of Jesus. Through prayer, we enforce the power of Jesus in our lives and in the lives and circumstances of those around us.

To the secular mind, this is unacceptable. There may come a point where one just has to try it to believe it. That is where one crosses the bridge to life beyond this physical existence.

CHAPTER 16

An Adoring Relationship

Once every four weeks I have an appointment to examine a herd of dairy cattle for their reproductive status. It is 1 p.m. on the second Monday of July. I just arrived at Ben's farm to examine his herd of about 100 Holstein dairy cows. Ben is usually not present for the examinations. Instead, he has a hired hand to accompany me as I examine the cows.

Lud is an elderly man. His face is tired and worn. His clothing is dirty and ragged. The patches on his pants have worn holes in them. His clothing is so worn that it is borderline indecent. He does not have a beard but clearly needs a shave. He walks with a stiff and painful limp. His knees are worn out. It comes from the constant standing and squatting from years of milking cows in a tie stall barn. Lud is here today as he always is every four weeks to assist me.

As I enter the barn, I see Lud. He is where he always is upon my arrival. He is lying on a blanket spread across two hay bales along the side of the barn. He appears to be sound asleep, but I know the routine. As he hears me enter the barn, he opens one eye ever so slightly to see me. I catch his glance. As soon as our eyes meet, he firmly closes both eyes and begins to snore, a fake snore.

Cuddled beside Lud on the bales is a small beagle dog. His name is Spud. Spud is nothing special. He is a mutt. He is dirty like Lud. His eyes show his age. They are cloudy from the cataracts of age. Lud and Spud are inseparable. Wherever Lud goes, Spud goes.

I do not know where Lud lives. He is always asleep on the

bales when I arrive at the farm. I suspect that Lud and Spud live in the barn along with all the cows. He does not have any friends or family. The other workers on the farm tease him and make fun of him. His life is lonely and bitter. He is usually complaining about someone or something. It is apparent that his comments arise from the hurt within him. The only friend he has is Spud. Spud is loyal and adoring of crusty old Lud. Spud's soft, cloudy eyes glow when he looks up at Lud. When Lud returns the soft gaze, he does so with a smile and a few soft words. Lud speaks lovingly of Spud.

I begin examining cows with Lud. As I examine each cow and report to Lud, he writes down the diagnosis on a worn-out notebook. The pages are torn but still usable. This is rather boring so I strike up a conversation with Lud. Farming and the weather are interrelated. I talk about the nice warm weather of today. Lud complains that it is too cold.

This starts a long list of complaints emanating from the hurts within Lud. I have known Lud for many years. I make a point of not aggravating him. I am just a good listener. I resign myself to examining cows and listening to Lud's complaints. His complaints go in one ear and out the other. Spud is at Lud's side and just seems grateful to be near Lud. He is loyal to Lud no matter what happens.

It took over an hour to complete the exams. As I wrap up my visit, I say a gentle goodbye and I will see you again in four weeks.

"Lud, have a nice day."

Lud softens up a bit as he returns the goodbye and reaches down to place a gentle, adoring pat on Spud's head. Lud and Spud are best friends. The two of them need each other because they only have each other.

A few years later on a hot July day I went to Ben's farm and Lud was not there. Spud was not there either. Both were gone. I learned that a few days earlier in the midst of a very hot day,

Lud had collapsed in the barn. They found him lying on the dirty floor, deceased. I do not know anything else about family, friends, and acquaintances. I do not even know if there was any type of service to remember his life. Moreover, I do not know what happened to Spud.

Lud and Spud's relationship demonstrates what people desire within themselves. They desire an inward security that comes from experiencing a relationship not based upon performance. It remains in spite of the inevitable disappointments, personal failures, and troubles life hands us. Everyone needs to know that their life has value. They need to know that they belong. They need a friend that accepts them for who they are no matter what they have or have not done. Life is lonely without such a friend.

People are by nature competitive. They may compare themselves to one another. They elevate themselves by degrading others. This leads to hurt and rejection. They give up on relationships with other people. They harbor anger as they lead a lonely and bitter life. They have no one to turn to for the security of a true friendship because they fear more rejection.

They look to the comforts of this world for a place to belong. They will try expensive materialism, drugs, addictions, stardom, and the acquisition of power and wealth. They are searching but nothing seems to be a long-term solution to the emptiness within them. It is a downward spiral out of control. The emptiness remains and intensifies.

In the search for that inward security, people throughout history have created religions to fill that inward space. The unique aspect of the Christian God is that He revealed Himself to us by coming to us as one of us in the person of Jesus. He came to us. We did not create Him. In fact, when He came to us, many rejected Him because He was different than what people expected. Nevertheless, His influence on mankind has endured the ages.

When one accepts the existence of a spiritual reality, it opens up a whole new possibility for such a relationship. Jesus Christ proclaimed the existence of a spiritual reality. His life with us demonstrated the spiritual reality beyond our physical existence.

Jesus claimed to be the bread of life. He claimed to be living water. It seems ridiculous for someone to claim to be bread and water. He used the examples of the need for bread and water to sustain our physical bodies as an example of the need for knowing Jesus to sustain our spiritual lives. Bread and water are to our physical bodies as Jesus is to our spiritual bodies. He promises to never reject or abandon us once we invite Him inward as a friend.

As time passes us by, our physical lives on this earth will vanish just as it did for Lud and Spud. However, time is just another dimension in the physical world. The spiritual world is not constrained by the dimension of time. As such, it is eternal. It does not end. God is eternal. He is timeless. He always has been and always will be. He came to earth as a human in the person of Jesus. His message was that there is much more to reality than just your physical existence. Jesus' life is God reaching out to people to restore a relationship with them. If we accept that as a truth, His spirit resides within us as a friend. He promises to stay with us through whatever this life throws at us. Moreover, it is timeless, forever, in the spiritual realm.

The first step is to acknowledge that there is at least a possibility of the reality of a spiritual existence. Once our minds are open to that possibility, we see life in an entirely different way. We see the interaction of the spiritual with the physical. We see the realities of good and evil in both the physical and spiritual realms.

It fosters a desire to know more. It starts a search to discover the truth about spirituality, God, Jesus, and the biblical record. Are they just stories and tales told through the centuries by dreaming minds? On the other hand, are they true?

The growing belief in the spiritual is bolstered by ancient prophesies that are fulfilled with accuracy centuries later. Compared to all other religions, this is a unique aspect of Christianity. There are too many of them to be purely coincidental. It becomes more reasonable to believe in the existence of a spiritual reality and of God coming as the person of Jesus to retrieve lost people than to not believe.

We start by admitting that we cannot be perfectly good by our own efforts. The inward life is that secret awareness of who we really are. It is where our spontaneous unspoken thoughts come from. One can know who they really are by examining those thoughts. No one else sees or hears it unless we show or tell them. It is the spirit within us. It can be for good or for evil. There are plenty of examples throughout human history of both. It is ours to decide which we want to pursue.

As we examine our inner thoughts and desires, we discover our real motives. We discover unspoken evil within those motives. It shakes our confidence in our desire to be good. Most people do not let those thoughts lead to actions. They rightly repress those thoughts. However, the very presence of those unwholesome thoughts within us reveals an underlying sinful nature.

We have a choice. We can continue life in denial of a spiritual existence even though it keeps resurfacing in our minds. If we continue in that denial, the conflict within our minds leads to disappointment in ourselves. It leads to an inner turmoil and unhappiness. That leads to a determination to do better and to stop those unwholesome thoughts. No matter how hard we try to do better, the unwholesomeness eventually resurfaces. We vacillate in conflict between the good and the bad. Specific instances of our failures come to our mind as regrets and sorrow.

The alternative is to admit that we cannot overcome the

conflict by our own resolve. The conflict is a spiritual battle. We need to fight that battle in the spiritual realm, not the physical realm. It starts with remorse in admitting that we have failed. Repentance is deep sorrow or contrition for a past wrongdoing.

At this point one must consider the life of Jesus. He said He was the Son of Man and the Son of God. He was God come to us as a human to reveal to us our need for God. He told us that we are not perfect. We cannot help but mess up our lives. He called it sin. We all have that trait. It separates us from knowing God. God deplores sin but not the sinner. We can try to be perfect on our own effort but we will fail.

God wants us back. That requires a sacrifice to right the wrongs we have done and will do. God did not explain why he requires a sacrifice. He only said that it does require a sacrifice. Many cultures have performed sacrifices to please their gods. Some of them were quite brutal and disgusting. The Mayans of Central America and the Incas of South America would conduct human sacrifices including children. It seems that the idea was to use a substitution to right the wrongs of the guilty ones before their gods.

Before the life of Jesus, the Judaic sacrifice was in the form of animals or grains. Then God sent Jesus to reveal His desire to be present in our inner lives. Jesus' physical time among us culminated in His own mortal death as a sacrifice for the sin of all people. Ancient prophesy foretold His sacrifice long before it occurred (Isaiah 52:13-53:12, Psalm 22:16-18).

Jesus' physical life was not terminated by the crucifixion. He returned to the living by His resurrection. This, too, was prophesied a thousand years before it happened (Psalm 16:9-10) and by Jesus himself before His crucifixion (Matthew 12:40). His promise before the crucifixion was to return as a new presence in the form of the Holy Spirit in the hearts of all who believe in Christ (John 14:15-17). The prophet Ezekiel (Ezekiel 37:14) also prophesied this 600 years before Christ.

He now lives among those who choose to accept Him into their inner life by the presence of the Holy Spirit. If we desire to enter that spiritual reality, we do so by inviting Jesus to be our inward life.

The life of Christ and the sequence of events from His birth to the resurrection are so unnatural to our concepts of physical life that they are hard to believe. One can only conclude that if they are true, then Jesus was far more than just another good person. As the centurion filled with awe at the events accompanying Jesus' crucifixion said, "Truly this was the Son of God" (Mathew 27:54).

If one rejects these events, then they must reject the unmistakable reality and accuracy of prophesies recorded centuries before they occurred.

What difference does the presence of the Holy Spirit make in a person? It does not mean we become perfect. It means that we have an inner friend that helps guide our way in the pathway of life. We still have our good days and bad days. The friend within brings us to an ability to deal with ourselves. We are encouraged in the good times. We come to repentance and dismissal of our bad times in place of a downward spiral of frustration and disappointment. We acquire an inner voice that encourages us to choose the good and brings us to a resolution of dealing with the bad. Our motives are directed toward love, joy, peace, patience, kindness, goodness, faithfulness, gentleness, and self-control (Galatians 5:22).

CHAPTER 17

A Special Friend

"You were made by God and for God.
Until you understand that, life will never make sense."
- Rick Warren

I grew up on a dairy farm. Dairy farms require a lot of hard work from everyone in the family. Cows need to be fed, milked, and kept clean and comfortable every day of their life. I will always treasure those formative years and I am thankful for the life, work ethic, and values that my parents instilled in me on the farm. I can still remember the names of some of my favorite dairy cows. Cows are docile, curious, yet shy creatures. They will cautiously approach you to investigate you with their nose. As soon as they touch you, they will back away in a shy manner. If you gain their trust, they will allow you to be near them and to pet them.

Small family dairy farms were abundant when I entered my profession as a veterinarian. On any specific farm, I got to know all members of the family including the father, mother, children, dogs, and even some special cows. I became part of their world in a limited way. I was granted the privilege of being part of their relationship with their cows.

On one such farm, I got to know a young boy named Alex. Most kids love animals. Alex was no different and he had a special cow that was his friend. Her name was Daisy. Daisy gave birth to a bouncing, healthy heifer days ago but now was feeling ill. I receive a call to come out to the farm to examine, diagnose, and treat her.

Upon arrival at the farm, I receive the usual greeting by a friendly Labrador retriever, named Grover. Grover likes Milk Bone treats. He strategically places himself at my feet, sits down, and looks at me patiently with those smiling but pleading eyes.

I have no choice but to comply with Grover's reception. "Ok, Grover, here's your treat. But you only get one." He gulps it down almost whole without chewing it. I often wondered how he knew it tastes so good when he seems to swallow the treat whole. There is very little contact with his taste buds.

I enter the barn and Alex is there waiting for me. He is very concerned. Daisy is ill. She does not eat anything and if left in this condition, she will die. She needs to regain her appetite to and be a productive member of the family. Daisy needs medical help or Alex will lose his friend.

As I examine her, I determine that she has a common condition called ketosis. It occurs after calving because there is a sudden increase in energy demand brought on by the metabolic demands of calving and the onset of lactation.

I retrieve the medicines that I need to treat her for this condition from my car. I secure her head with a halter, place an IV in her jugular vein, and start the IV drip of dextrose. This is a slow process.

Alex is a talkative little guy and so we start to chat. He tells me about the details of Daisy's life. She is 4 years old. This is the second calf she has delivered. Both are heifers. The first one is named Donna and this one will be named Duchess. She is a big eater and eats anything placed in front of her. She gives a lot of milk, often over 12 gallons per day. Her favorite food is cheesesteaks.

"What!" I proclaim. "She eats cheesesteaks. Doesn't she eat hay, grass, silage, and grains like all the other cows?"

"Yes she likes those but my favorite food is cheesesteaks and when mom makes cheesesteaks for our meals I always bring one out to the barn for Daisy. She loves them. We eat them together."

"Ok," I say with a grin as I finish treating Daisy. "Hopefully she'll get back up to par and start eating this afternoon. Are you having cheesesteaks for dinner?"

"I don't know but I'll put in a request for cheesesteaks for dinner."

These kinds of relationships add spice to my profession. Every day is an adventure. You never know what may come your way on any given day. Never in my wildest dreams did I ever expect to come across a cheesesteak-eating cow.

Alex and Daisy have a special unspoken relationship. Alex knows what Daisy likes and it is his delight to provide for her.

When one comes to accept a spiritual reality, they become a seeker of the truths that occupy that space. Throughout human history, cultures have instinctively celebrated spiritual traditions. Some have been based upon love and compassion and some have been quite violent, manifesting the existence of good and evil. Good and evil are themes that occupy much of our literature, theater, politics, and religions. The truth is that humans have within them an awareness of their spiritual nature and the existence of good and evil in both the natural and spiritual worlds.

Whatever one believes about the origin of life, the truth is that it originated from God. God created life for His own purpose. His purpose is for good. As the timeline of His creation moved along, He desired for a higher life form in that creation to possess a likeness of God Himself, a spiritual likeness. He gave people a spiritual possession in His own image. It was for good and it was good.

God's intent is for humans to be aware of His presence in their lives. He wants to be in a relationship with people. Like Alex and Daisy, God wants to know and interact with people. He also gave humans the freedom to make choices. It is God's delight for people to independently choose to be in a relationship with God. They did just that, for a time.

However, because they had freedom to choose, they decided to be gods themselves. Evil crept into their lives and became an inherent part of their nature.

God wants us back. It is our decision. His delight is to be with us in a spiritual relationship. We are made by God and for God. Once we gain that awareness, our priorities and values change for the good.

CHAPTER 18

The Tornado

Grandchildren are a delight. At a young age, they are ador-ing and so impressionable. As a grandfather, one just wants to establish a good relationship with them and make good impressions on them. What better way to do that then to spend time with them and allow them to see you at work and at play.

It is my weekend on call for our veterinary practice. It is a warm day, especially for the middle of February. What a nice foretaste of summer as the air temperature is into the seventies. I receive a call from a longtime client that he has a sick cow and he suspects that she has a displaced abomasum, or as we say, a DA. I travel to the farm with my car windows partly open just enjoying the mild weather. After examining the cow, I confirm that she indeed does have a DA and needs surgery to correct it.

Previously, my son-in-law has said that he wants to see what I do and that if there was ever an opportunity to watch me at work he would like that and he would bring my grand-son along so that the two of them could have a bonding ex-perience. I call Joe to see if he wants to come watch with his young 4-year-old son, Isaac. He eagerly agreed and brought Isaac along to the farm for the two of them to witness their first surgery on a dairy cow. It is a nice reason to get outside on a beautiful warm day in the midst of the dreariness and gray of most winter days.

As they watch, I set up my operating room in a small box stall in the barn next to the outside feed bunk where the cows eat their feed rations. As I do my surgical prep on the cow, I notice dark clouds beginning to form in the western sky. It's February and the weather can change quickly. The cloud grows bigger and darker as I continue with the procedure.

My audience watches closely as I make my incision and begin the surgery. I begin to become somewhat concerned about the impending weather as the barn is open on the side-walls and greatly exposed to the outside conditions. The wind begins to blow and it is obvious that a storm is about to break out all around us. I am committed to the procedure now. I ignore the storm and continue the task. I proceed to the most critical part of the surgery where I expose the stomach and se-cure it in the proper location.

Suddenly there is a terrific blast of wind. It begins to rain. The wind howls and the rain becomes very heavy, com-ing down in sheets just a few feet from me outside of the ex-posed building. It is raining so hard that a river of water flows through the barn as water runs off from the outside paved area. Hail pounds down on the roof above me with a deafening roar. The cows that are outside panic and stampede for shelter wher-ever they could find it. The wind and rain howl even more. It sounds like a freight train. I have no choice but to focus on the task. I continue with the surgery while the wind is howling and the drenching rain is creating rivers of water around me.

I glance at Joe who is usually cool and calm. He, too, is quite concerned. We all are. I hope the barn does not blow away. I hope that if it does no one will be injured. That seems like a distinct possibility. Young Isaac buries his head in his dad's shoulder and clings to Joe for protection. At the height of the storm, danger is quite imminent. I tell them to go to a more secure area of the barn away from the wind and water. What have I done? I have brought family into a dangerous situation. What seemed like a great opportunity for a bonding family event has turned into a disaster.

As I begin to wrap up the final aspects of the procedure

the wind dies down, the rain stops, and in a few minutes, the sun breaks through the clouds and a tranquil but much cooler February day resumes. I later learn that a tornado touched down only a few miles to the east of our location. Apparently, it had passed over our location. My good intentions to make a favorable impression on these dear members of my family are washed away with the terror of the storm.

I had good intentions. I had good plans. Nevertheless, it was not to be. It is a theme of human nature to place our confidence in our own desires and abilities. Our culture encourages us to be confident in ourselves, to go our own way. Often no harm results. Sometimes though it leads to calamity and to conflicts with grave consequences. The desire to serve selfish interests has led to wars and mass exterminations of people.

What would life on this earth be like if there was a supreme being, a God that guided everyone's thoughts and actions for the good of all mankind? People would tune into God for guidance before actions. People would be directed to desire the common good of all above their own desires and ambitions for wealth and power.

People would seek to hear the voice of God in their thoughts before taking instinctive actions that benefit themselves at the expense of those around them. Our lives are not there, yet. No one perfectly meets that challenge. Many try but ultimately fail.

God offers that guidance. He understands the depravity of our own desires. He offers to provide a source of guidance within ourselves that directs our thoughts and actions for our own good and the greater good. It is a voice in our thoughts originating from the Holy Spirit.

The clarity of that voice can be confused by thoughts that are not from God. There is a continual battle within our thoughts of good vs. evil. Decisions that we make reflect the outcome of that battle. The thoughts precede the actions.

Life is a progression of seeking to hear that voice clearly without the confusion of the wrong voice. We never get it right all the time. We are born with that nature. We have a choice to make. If we choose the wrong voice, it leads to bad things happening.

God made us to be in a relationship with Him. We drifted from that relationship to go our own self-directed way.

He wants us back. He came as a human, Jesus, to provide a way for us to return to Him every time we get it wrong and fail. Jesus' message to the world is that there is a spiritual kingdom not of this physical world. Throughout His life, He proclaims that His Kingdom is not of this world. He came to open our eyes to a spiritual reality. He came to show us the depravity of following our own desires in contrast to hearing God's voice. He said that He never did anything without first hearing God's instruction. This is the model for us to follow as we accept the reality of God and the spiritual conflict within ourselves.

When we accept that Spiritual reality, we gain a different understanding of the conflicts we encounter. The conflicts, struggles, disappointments, and hardships of life that we encounter are still there. We see their origin in the spiritual. We fight our battles in the spiritual realm through prayer before we take actions in the physical realm. God is there to guide us through those battles as we choose to seek His voice through the Holy Spirit.

CHAPTER 19

A Testing of My Faith

"We see things not as they are, but as we are."
- H. M. Tomlinson

I learned to appreciate the sport of soccer when I was at recess in elementary school where one of the teachers organized impromptu soccer games at every recess. I later played on a start-up high school team and continued in college. When my kids were old enough to play, I coached their teams for many years. I will never regret those years. They allowed me to be a part of my kids' lives and to know their friends as well.

Team sports teach us about the ups and downs of life. Sometimes you win and sometimes you lose. Losing can be more important than winning as it builds character and teaches us how to deal with disappointment. Losing builds stamina. Never give up. Pull yourself back up off the ground and keep going. Try harder.

Winning is the reward for hard work. However, do not assume that you are entitled to it. A team can play at the top of their game, controlling the ball with finesse, precise passing, working the ball through the defense for an awesome shot upper ninety on the goal, which bounces off the crossbar. A few inches lower and it is a score. You play the whole game easily outperforming your opponent and then lose 1-0 from a fluke goal scored by your outplayed opponent who went unnoticed in an offside position. One mistake cost you the whole game.

My daughter and her friends were on several middle school teams that I coached. We were competitive with other teams in our age group and grew together as a team of players and supportive parents as we traveled to games and tournaments.

It is said that defense wins games. Build a great defense, keep the ball in your opponent's half of the field and the goals will come. The sweeper is the last player on defense before the goalkeeper. The sweeper will work with the defense to break up scoring opportunities from the opposing team.

In one particular game, our team was shorthanded as some players had other commitments that day. The girl who played the sweeper position was away for the day. She was an awesome all-around player that could play any position. I played her at the critical sweeper position.

The youngest girl on our team was quiet and shy. Jennie was very athletic. She played as an outside defensive back. She was tall and ran like a gazelle, fast and graceful. Since our regular sweeper was away, I decided to try Jennie at the sweeper position. She had a fantastic game. When the game was over, parents and players alike marveled at how she had played the position. In that one game, Jennie proved her ability to play sweeper. She had made the most of the opportunity. She played sweeper for us the rest of that season and the seasons to follow. Jennie was fantastic.

We practice twice a week, Tuesdays and Thursdays, with games on Sunday afternoon. I organize the practices in a format that consists of starting with some conditioning and stretching. Then we move onto practicing individual ball skills, followed by short-sided games, and eventually move onto scrimmages. I always include a portion of the practice that involves taking shots on goal. Everyone wants to score goals and so this is a favorite part of practices.

It is a Tuesday evening practice. The team is shooting on goal with the aim of scoring in the side netting of the goal.

The idea is to encourage players to place their shots away from where the goalkeeper can make an easy save. Players line up behind the eighteen-yard line, receive a crossing pass from me, and take a one-touch shot on goal. It is going well as shots challenge both the shooter and the goalkeeper.

Jennie is up next. She starts her run on goal, I pass her the ball and she shoots on goal. As she completes her run, she collapses in the mouth of the goal. I run over to her as she lay on the ground. I am a veterinarian. My experience with biological life tells me immediately that her life is in trouble. I recognize the signs of life leaving her. This is no trip over the ball incident. She needs immediate medical attention.

My assistant coaches start CPR. Parents call 911. There is a medical office next to our field. Instinctively, I immediately run to that office and tell them I have a player that has collapsed on the field and needs immediate medical attention. To their credit, they recognize the seriousness in my voice and a doctor and nurse hurriedly come immediately with me to the field where Jennie lie motionless. They continue the CPR until an EMS medical unit arrives. She is still unresponsive.

As the medical technicians care for Jennie, the concern for Jennie grows. By now, other teams notice the emergency activity and as practices end, many other players came from other fields to our practice field.

As word spreads, players and coaches form a large circle and start impromptu prayers for Jennie, asking God to intervene on behalf of Jennie.

Jennie's parents are not at the practice. I make a call to them to inform them that Jennie has collapsed at practice and is on her way to the hospital. I go to the hospital to meet them. I just need to know how Jennie is doing. I arrive in the waiting area of the emergency room before her parents. They arrive and I introduce them to the receptionist.

They are taken to Jennie. As I wait for what seems like

an eternity there is no word about Jennie's condition. I need to know. I just wait. Eventually, her parents come back to the waiting area. Their faces show the seriousness of her condition. They tell me that Jennie is still unconscious. The only thing that can be done now is to wait to see how she progresses.

I promised to tell the rest of the team a report from the hospital. I call everyone on the team to inform them of Jennie's condition. I go home but do not sleep that night. It is a night where you are exhausted but sleep does not come. The visual images of traumatic events never leave your mind. With time, the emotion fades but the images are there for a lifetime.

That morning, as every morning, I read the local newspaper. I find a front-page article on Jennie. No more details on her condition are given. That day I go about my work. I cannot get Jennie out of my mind. I just exist as best I can to meet the challenges of the day.

Prayer chains are alerted throughout the area. It seems that there is an army of prayers going up on Jennie's behalf. It occurs to me that this is an opportunity for God to show Himself to many people young and old. With so many young impressionable minds at the soccer field that are aware of what has happened, this is a divine opportunity for God to manifest His healing power and bring Jennie back to us.

The next few days fill with uncertainty and little new information. I pray often, confident in knowing that this is God's opportunity to turn hearts towards Him. I insist upon that.

I take up the spiritual weapons we are granted in Ephesians 6:12. "For our struggle is not against flesh and blood, but against the rulers, against the authorities, against the powers of this dark world and against the spiritual forces of evil in the heavenly realms."

I fight the battle for Jennie in the heavenly realm. I am not going to let the enemy of God and His people take her from us.

As the days pass with little word of her condition, I continue the spiritual battles. Five days pass. It is Sunday evening. We gather as a team and parents. I do not want to give up hope. Jennie is still unconscious but stable on life support. A parent that is a nurse at the hospital warns me of her grave condition. I will have none of it. I do not want to accept that as an outcome. I am confident that God will come through. Do not let this young 13-year-old innocent girl be taken from this life.

As we are still gathered together, I receive a call from Jennie's parents at the hospital. Jennie has passed away and they are donating her organs to others in need of the blessing of life. Her physical life on earth has ended.

That next week is a time of great grief. Jennie's funeral is filled with her teammates, friends, classmates, parents, friends of parents, and many people who come to show that they care. I serve as a pallbearer. It is an honor. It also emphasizes the finality of her condition.

My thoughts are confused. It is an inward struggle. I expected God to fulfill my desire. It would seem that would be His desire as well. I struggle with God. I feel abandoned by Him. I do not feel love.

It is the following Sunday again, one week after Jennie died. I go to church as usual. As the congregation gathers in worship, the words of the songs become impossible for me to sing. I just stand there, stunned. I cannot sing these songs. I am tired of the rhetoric. God did not come through as I had wanted and prayed. I was furious. God, You want us to worship You and You treat us like this!

My anger festered. I know I need to deal with it. I had too many good encounters with God that I could not deny Him. Yet I was angry with Him. Friends noticed. They were caring and gracious with kind words and support. Some gave me books. I sought books that were meant to explain why God does not always answer prayers the way we want Him to answer them. I read them. Book after book just gave a list of excuses for God. I had no answers to my predicament. The anger remained.

I went back to God demanding an explanation. He did not provide one. He does not owe us an explanation. The one thing that He did tell me was that it is OK to be angry with Him. That rather surprised me because I was also feeling guilty for daring to be angry with God Almighty. How presumptuous is that? He told me that being angry means we have a relationship. One does not get angry with someone they could care less about. He comforted me in my struggle. It was good to hear from Him.

I remember that when my father was abruptly taken in a farm accident, a wise old veterinarian told me that it takes two years of grieving to overcome the loss. Those were wise words. I existed for at least two years struggling to get answers. With time, the emotion faded and I was able to think beyond my emotions. I still had no answers acceptable to me. I gave up in my struggle to find answers. I came to the end of being able to figure it out for myself. I still needed something in my mind to settle the issue.

It was in that state of being at the end of myself and my abilities to understand, that God came to me with a simple answer. "I am God and you are not God. I see events in the perspective of eternity. Some things are beyond your comprehension. There are things that you will not understand. Be still and know that I am God."

It is not the understanding that I wanted. Nevertheless, it is an answer that with time, I understand. God is omnipotent. He is infinite. He is the source of all that is true. He is the source of everything that is in existence. He is timeless. He always has been. He always will be. He made the laws of physics. He made the laws that govern the universe. The sun rises every day. It sets every evening. I do not control any of that. He does. I do not understand much of that either.

Who am I to demand an explanation from the maker of the universe? Many things are beyond my finite ability to understand. This event is something I will never understand in this life. So while I do not have an answer, I do understand. God's ways are higher than my ways. He sees everything in its entirety. I only see in part. So be it. I will rest in knowing that I will not understand this one. I am limited by my own expectations. I see things as I am, not necessarily as they are. Only God sees things as they really are—past, present, and future—all in one time frame.

Everyone we meet is afraid of something, loves someone or something, and has lost someone or something. We expect God to be the great "fixer upper." We expect Him to make our lives trouble free and perfect. We want to be winners.

Yet life is full of losing. When I encounter hardship, I desire for God to "fix it." Instead, He will walk through that hardship with me. As I reflect back on Jennie, I can see that in spite of my anger and struggle with God, He did not discard me. He patiently walked with me to bring me to a place where I could let go of my expectations. He brought me to a place of humility in accepting what I could not initially accept. I learned that God is God and I am not God.

CHAPTER 20

Mortality

*"Not everything that counts can be counted,
and not everything that can be counted counts."*
- Albert Einstein

Death is a subject we do not like to consider. Yet at some point, we all will face it. It is inevitable. For some people the very thought of facing it is terrifying. Others seek it perhaps to their own demise. Some are fascinated, almost preoccupied with studying it. Some just accept the inevitability of death and attempt to live every day to its fullest, either for their interest or to better the lives of those around them.

It brings up the subject of why does life exist in the first place if it must end. When one considers the vast expanse of the universe, why do we even exist? We know of no other celestial body where life as we know it exists. Is life just a cosmic accident based upon the laws of probability? Given the odds of something happening, it just happened.

When one becomes aware of the complexity of living organisms, the odds of life just happening are infinitesimally small, perhaps impossible. In a closed system, the state of disorder increases. A system only becomes more organized if an outside force enters to increase the state of order within the system. That is what has happened with the existence of life.

This planet went from a state of chaos and disorder to a

more organized state of abundant life forms as we know them. The ultimate question though is why did it happen? What outside force was applied to the system to increase the orderliness that is the existence of life within this system? Some call that evolution. Others call it creation by God. Evolution alone though would still require the application of an outside force to increase the degree of order within the system. However, all the individual physical bodies of these life forms still lose their orderliness. They age, become diseased, pass away and decay. Ashes to ashes and dust to dust.

There once was a man that said the forms of life we consider the most advanced, people, can live forever. As time passes their physical bodies will erode and decay, but something within them can live forever.

From the very beginning of our existence, people have sought to understand this inner something. People throughout history have sought a spiritual reality. They have sought immortality. The creation account in Genesis tells us that people are created in the image of God. God is a spiritual reality. People have within them a spiritual reality.

The man's name was Jesus. His amazing life is recorded in the Bible. His existence was prophesized in ancient manuscripts written centuries before His life. The beyond natural occurrences of His life were foretold of centuries before they occurred.

Jesus said that He came to us to tell us about the truth. John 14:6a "I am the way and the truth and the life."

He told us that we are not perfect. He told us that we all have fallen away from God's intention for us. Romans 3:23 "for all have sinned and fall short of the glory of God."

He told us that there is a cosmic conflict between good and evil. Mathew 13:38 "The field is the world, and the good seed stands for the people of the kingdom. The weeds are the people of the **evil** one."

God told us in the Old Testament that sin separates us from God. Isaiah 59:2 "But your iniquities have separated you from your God; your sins have hidden his face from you."

Jesus tells us that He is sent to us by God. John 8:42 "Jesus said to them, 'If God were your Father, you would love me, for I have come here from God. I have not come on my own; God sent me.'"

He is sent to release us from the consequence of sin. Romans 6:23 "For the wages of sin is death, but the gift of God is eternal life in Christ Jesus our Lord."

Jesus tells us that God desires for us to live eternally with Him in the spirit. John 6:40 "For my Father's will is that everyone who looks to the Son and believes in Him shall have eternal life."

He tells us that there is only one way to reach that spiritual life with God and that is through Jesus. John 14:6b "No one comes to the Father except through me."

He told us that the supernatural works He did were to testify that He is sent to us by God. John 5:36 "For the works that the Father has given me to finish—the very works that I am doing—testify that the Father has sent me."

Jesus also told us that for us to know eternal spiritual life, He must go through the death and resurrection we know as Easter. Mark 8:31 "He then began to teach them that the Son of Man must suffer many things and be rejected by the elders, the chief priests and the teachers of the law, and that He must be killed and after three days rise again."

Mortality refers to the inevitable demise of our physical bodies. Yet Jesus offers us immortality, to live forever. God created us to be in a spiritual relationship with Him. That worked for a while, but eventually mankind abandoned that relationship and cut ties with God. We departed from that spiritual relationship with God.

God wants us back. Jesus is sent by God to restore our relationship with God. Each person needs to earnestly seek truth in the life of Jesus rather than dismiss Him as a fantasy. Do not accept popular culture. Engage your own search for truth. If a person accepts the reality of Jesus into their life, they overcome mortality through spiritual immortality.

Jesus at the cross is the bridge between our physical body and the spiritual reality that humans have sought to encounter throughout their history. God used the cross to provide a path for us to know Him intimately and to be the dwelling place of His Holy Spirit. There is only one bridge available to all who choose to look for the other side. Because of the life and crucifixion of Jesus, the physical body of a human animal can harbor the Spirit of God.

As we meditate on the events of Easter let us conclude with a prayer.

Our Father in Heaven, hallowed be thy name. Thy Kingdom come, Thy will be done on earth as it is heaven. Father God, we are in awe of You. You are the creator of life, the one who put it all together. You desire to know each of us personally, in the spiritual realm. Your desire is for us to reach beyond our mundane existence and discover life in You. We acknowledge our sinful existence. We are not worthy of Your presence. We have fallen to self-indulgence and the pride of self-righteousness. Forgive us our sins as we forgive those who sin against us. Please lead us not into temptation but deliver us from the evil one. As the world around us crumbles, turn our focus to You and away from the entrapments of grabbing power and fame for our own benefit. Thank You so much for Your gracefulness in caring for us by sending Jesus to bring truth to our awareness of You. Thanks for His obedience to pay the price for our redemption. Thank You for Jesus and His sacrifice for us. Thank You for providing the Holy Spirit to us today to help us know You. Sharpen that inner voice of the Holy Spirit. Grant us the ears to hear. Make us aware of the conflicts between good and evil that are before us. Guard us from the deception the enemy places before us.

Let us not fall into apathy but rather take up the sword of the spirit to destroy the work of the enemy in our midst. Thank You for the promise of eternal life in You. Without Jesus, we would surely die. With Jesus, we graduate to a higher realm. For Yours is the kingdom, the power, and the glory forever and ever. It is only because of Jesus that we can come to You. Amen.

CHAPTER 21

What Difference Does It Make?

Stephen has a small herd of 40 cows. He knows them as individuals. Each cow has a name he has given them at birth. He knows each cow's life story, her extended family, and her strengths and weaknesses. His experience guides him in helping each cow benefit from their strengths and overcome their weaknesses. The cows do not know it but he is their advocate.

It is about noon on a bright and very hot summer Sunday afternoon. I am on call. I am on my way home from church. I receive a text on my work phone. Stephen has a cow that has lacerated her milk vein and is bleeding profusely. Please come ASAP.

I recognize the emergency. The milk vein is a large vein that runs along the underside of a cow covered only by a thin layer of skin. It is about the size of a garden hose and carries a large volume of blood from the udder back to the heart.

About five percent of body weight is blood. A 1,600-pound cow will have about 10 gallons of blood in her body. Because this vein is so large, a cow can lose a lot of blood volume quickly if the vessel is lacerated. Time is critical. In fact, if Stephen does not do something to stop the flow of blood before I arrive, the cow will lose so much blood that I will not be able to save her life. The scene is usually a bloody mess. My task will be to locate the laceration and ligate the vein to stop the flow of blood.

I arrive at the farm. I am in my dress clothing. I can see that the family is in the barn with Stephen and the cow. I

141

quickly go to the milk house and discreetly change into work clothing, hoping no one notices.

I enter the barn to find Stephen under the cow pressing his hand against the milk vein to stop the bleeding. There is a large clot of blood around him. Stephen is sweating profusely. His clothing is wet and soaked with dark blood. Sweat is pouring from his forehead. He struggles to keep his hand placing pressure over the laceration. His position crouched under the cow is awkward. He is vulnerable to injury. The cow could weaken and fall on him. She could resist his presence and kick him. He is exhausted but refuses to give up the battle against the hemorrhage.

His family surrounds him to cheer him on. Apparently, Stephen was bringing his cows back into the barn from the bright and hot sun in the pasture to protect them from the heat of the day. He has fans in the barn to cool the cows.

This cow's name is Ruth. Ruth slipped and fell on a sharp object. When she got back up, blood poured from underneath her body. She is an older cow. Her mammary veins are larger, more exposed, and more susceptible to injury than it would be for a younger cow.

I thank him for his wise decision to stop the bleeding before I arrived. I tell him to relax now and I will do my best to ligate the vein. He leaves his position from under the cow and as he does, blood again pours out from the laceration. It is everywhere. I cannot see anything because of all the blood.

Now I am sweating profusely. I take several large hemostats and begin clamping everywhere that I see opportunities to stop the flow. Finally, I am able to clamp off the vein and stop the hemorrhage. Thankfully, the cow has remained calm and upright. I can see the laceration. It is a clean cut through the large vein.

There is a blood clot all around it. I clean the clot away, clip the hair from around the laceration, and do a quick surgical scrub of the area with betadine scrub. Next, I inject an anesthetic around the area to desensitize it. This is tricky as the cow will feel the needle and may kick at me or knock the hemostats off the vein.

Stephen, now somewhat recovered from his ordeal, holds the cow's tail upright. This is an age-old trick to keep a cow distracted so that she is less likely to kick. We refer to it as "taking her out of gear" with a tail block. Sometimes I jokingly comment that cows have only one neuron. If we occupy that one neuron with the discomfort of a tail block, she is not aware of anything else.

Now that the area is desensitized, I am able to place several ligatures around the vein to stop the hemorrhage. I remove the hemostats and do a light surgical scrub to be sure there is no more bleeding. I examine Ruth's mucous membranes for a pink color and check her capillary refill as an indication of how much blood she has lost. Even though there is a red mess all around her, she will be fine.

Stephen's care for Ruth has saved her life. He stopped the flow before it became life ending. I merely plugged the leak. What difference does it make? His care for Ruth made a big difference in Ruth's life. Stephen intervened in Ruth's life to make a difference in Ruth's life.

What difference does having a spiritual relationship with God have in a person's life? What difference does not having such a relationship with God have in our lives? For many, our expectation is that our lives should be happy, carefree, and joyful.

When troubles or calamity enter one's life, as they inevitably will, our response can be one of fear, despair, and anger. We can feel isolated, alone, and overwhelmed. It can seem like the end. Often, our pride keeps us from reaching out for help and understanding from others. We do not want to admit that not all is well. We do not want to admit that we struggle. Yet we all do have times of calamity and struggle in our lives.

It would be great if there was a source within us that promises to never leave us, to always be present by our side, to never condemn, to make our burdens seem less stressful. The source within emerges as an inward knowing that is beyond our language and produces a calm confidence that rises up within us that somehow, someway, things will work out for our eventual good regardless of how bad it may seem now. It produces a hope that overcomes fear, anger, and despair.

Hope is something difficult to get our minds around. It is not something that is visible. Rather it is a state of mind. Yet it is what keeps us going from one day to the next. When hope is gone, despair prevails. Hope implies a better outcome. Despair implies a train wreck. It is hope that leads to courage, determination, and strength to meet the challenge.

We can source hope from material things, other people, events, or political ideologies. These sources of hope are short lived. They eventually fall short of our expectations because they arise from the entrapments of this physical world. They do not have a spiritual source. However, there is a spiritual reality. Its existence is not material, political, or circumstantial.

If we accept the concept of a spiritual reality and a spiritual aspect to our species, then God is a reality. He promises that if we enter into a relationship with Him through the revelations brought to us by Jesus, then He will always be part of our inward awareness. As we sincerely seek to be more aware of His promptings within us, He reveals more of Himself to us. He promises that there is nothing we have done, can do, or will do, that can separate us from Him. The promise is valid if we accept the life and teachings of Jesus as a means to come into a meaningful relationship with God.

So what difference does that make? The relationship with God as the Holy Spirit within us manifests as a hope that replaces despair. It manifests as a calm confidence in the midst of the storm. It manifests as courage instead of fear.

There is a knowing that life goes on in a different form when our physical bodies decay. It inspires courage to face our battles knowing that whatever the outcome may be, God will not abandon us. Just as Stephen stayed with Ruth through the life and death battle, so too God will stay with us.

It is a perspective on life that places a priority on knowing God in the spiritual realm above the trials, calamities, disappointments, job-related tasks, societal status, and expectations placed upon us by our society.

Much of our daily struggle is driven by our pride in being able to do it ourselves. We become dependent on that pride as a means of measuring our self-worth. That is a never-ending spiral into the trap of hopelessness.

Self-worth that comes from knowing there is a God that will stand with us sources hope from a relationship with God that gives us a perspective of life beyond this physical existence. It is a perspective that is more important than current events in our lives.

Knowing God in a day-by-day, minute-by-minute relationship does make a difference. It is a place where the grass is greener because it will arise from trusting that we have someone who is our advocate. The trials, pressures, and disappointments of each day becomes less important than an eternal perspective on life. There arises within us a sense of peace that in the end we will be alright. Where there is peace, there is joy. Where that joy surfaces, there is a desire to know God more and more every day. It is an upward spiral of joy. It replaces the downward spiral of pride that demolishes our self-worth through self-imposed disappointment.

CHAPTER 22

Battles

It is late afternoon on a cold dreary day in February. There is a light snow drifting to the ground. The air is thick with moisture. The high humidity makes the cold air penetrate to your bones. You feel a shiver up and down your backbone.

I have received a call late in the day to come to Joe's farm to examine a very sick cow. She delivered a calf early this morning.

Joe tells me she was fine this morning but has deteriorated during the day and now she will not eat anything and does not want to stand up. She is lying stretched out on her side in a stall. Her abdomen is distended with bloat.

Upon first seeing her, I suspect that she has milk fever. These cows appear very ill but respond very well to early treatment with intravenous calcium.

I go back to my car to retrieve the necessary equipment and medicines that I need for her treatment. As I leave through the barn door and round the corner of the barn to my car, I notice a cat on the hood of my car. As I get closer to my car, I notice another cat inside my car on the dashboard. Apparently, this cat entered my car through the open rear hatchback.

The two cats are howling at each other and are having a grand old tomcat battle. It is breeding season for cats. The tomcats are vying for dominance. There is one cat on the hood of my car and another cat inside my car on top of the dashboard. My windshield is between them. They see each other through my windshield and are angrily fighting each other. My windshield separates them and they become more and more frustrated as neither one of them can land any punches.

Tomcats mark their territory with urine. My windshield is splattered with tomcat urine inside and outside my car. These two cats are having a peeing contest. Tomcat urine is very pungent. The smell is suffocating.

I open the driver's door of my car and angrily evict the squatters from my car. They express their anger by hissing at me. They deposit one last spray of tomcat urine as they scurry away to resume the battle elsewhere. I will have a tomcat mess to clean up.

I have a cow to treat and for the moment, that is a priority. It is a routine task as I retrieve the necessary supplies and head back to the barn to treat the cow. The procedure goes smoothly and shortly after completing the treatment, the cow appears much better. She is now able to sit upright on her sternum and is relieving the bloat with voluminous belches. That is a great sound to hear in this situation.

I go back to my car and begin the malodorous task of cleaning up cat pee. It smells awful. I use strong soap and water with a towel to wipe down my dashboard, steering wheel, instrument panel, seats, floorboard, and the inside of the door. Finally, I have wiped down every surface with a strong-smelling soap to remove and cover up the odor.

I go back into the barn to check on the down cow. With a little urging, she rises to her feet. That is wonderful. I leave instructions for Joe to follow up with the cow so that her condition does not recur.

My task is completed. I wash up my boots and prepare to leave the farm. As I start up the car, I am rewarded with the horrific smell of cat pee directly into my face emanating from the defroster vents. Apparently, there are puddles of cat pee that have drained down into my defroster vents. They are beyond my reach. I drive home with the windows open and the heater and defroster on full blast during a dreary February snowstorm. For years to come I am reminded of this cat peeing contest every time I turn on the defroster. With time, the odor becomes fainter and bearable.

These cats fought a battle. I ran them off and the outcome was undecided. The damage was done. Their conflict continued until ultimately someone got hurt. It is the nature of battles. There are winners and losers. The outcome of this very physical battle will likely be determined by brute strength, agility, and perhaps feline pride.

People have battles to fight. Some are political wars beyond our control. Some are within our community or among our friends. We are bystanders for most of those battles. We have opinions but very little influence on their outcomes.

The battles that affect us in the most debilitating way are very personal conflicts. We listen to our thoughts. They condemn us for being so stupid and uncaring. How could I have said that to someone I care about? I should have stopped to help that person. Everyone hates me. They think very little of me. They laugh at me behind my back. I have no friends. No one will help me when I need it the most. They do not care if I disappear. In fact, they wish I would just leave. I am just going to withdraw and crawl in a hole. God hates me.

If we listen to these awful thoughts, we find ourselves in a very negative and destructive state of mind. These thoughts are lies. Where do these lies come from? They are a spiritual battle within us. There is a destructive spirit that desires to destroy what God has created. Satan is a liar that places those thoughts in our minds when we are most vulnerable.

It is an epic battle within us. We must recognize this as a spiritual battle. Recognize the source of those thoughts. Fight your battles first in the spiritual realm before you take an action. Rebuke the lies with the authority granted to those that know Jesus. Refuse to acknowledge them in any way. If there is one lie among all the accusations, then they are all lies.

Instead of listening to yourself, talk to yourself. Tell yourself that those thoughts are lies originating from an evil source. They are not welcome. I do not believe them. I am a unique creation of God with talents and gifting that God chose for me. Those talents and gifts will not be stifled by anyone or anything that chooses to elevate themselves by belittling me. I chose to follow the path God has placed on me. My confidence comes from God and not from myself.

For those that trust that God is on their side, they can take refuge in knowing that if they make the wrong decision, God promises not to abandon them. He will rescue them in spite of themselves.

It is here that a relationship with God, Jesus, and the Holy Spirit makes a difference. We still need to make decisions. We still need to consider the options and consequences. We trust there is a spiritual reality behind the scenes that has our long-term best interests as a priority. We can move ahead with our lives and not look back on our failures.

The most intense battles occur in the spiritual realm. Good and evil are very real forces among us. The conflicts we see in our physical world have an underlining spiritual battle behind the scenes. What we see in the physical world is the outcome of those spiritual battles. Failure to see where the real battle occurs leads to losing by default. Engaging the spiritual battle before the physical battle addresses the real source of the conflict.

It is in the spiritual battles that aligning with God through intense prayer and guidance from the Holy Spirit affects the outcome of those battles. It culminates in the physical reality for all to see. Before one engages a physical battle, win that battle in the spiritual realm through Holy Spirit directed prayer. That can only occur if there is already an established and nurtured relationship with God, Jesus, and the Holy Spirit.

The Holy Spirit promises to be our helper when we are so confused that we do not even know how to pray. I remember a prayer I had in the midst of a motorcycle accident. I had just been T-boned at an intersection by a car that did not stop for a stop sign. I was flying through the air and saw the grass whiz by underneath me. Before I made an ugly and painful landing, the only thought I had was a simple prayer: "God help me." It was not premeditated. It was just a prayer that came from within me when I needed it most. It was a Holy Spirit initiated prayer.

CHAPTER 23

He Knows Our Story

May is my favorite month of every year. I enjoy the springing forth of abundant new life in warmer weather. The grass is green and flowers are blooming. The birds are singing as they care for the little ones in their cozy nests. Beef cows are mooing over their newborn calves whom they tenderly nurse and care for as they roam about the plentiful fresh green grass. Fuzzy lambs follow their moms on lush green pastures. People seem to be more patient, including myself, as we are more relaxed in the warmer weather.

John is an elderly man that lives alone. He lives on a farm that shows years of gradual neglect as he ages alone. At a younger age, he was more attentive to the demands of maintenance of buildings and mowing of pastures on his farm. Now those demands have won the battle. His farm has decayed to the point of buildings in need of major repairs and pastures grown over with trees, briars, and weeds.

He calls this morning to ask if I will stop by his farm today to look at a sick beef cow. I thank him for the call and assure him that I will stop by either late morning or early afternoon. He is appreciative. John is a nice and gentle guy. Some call him a hermit because he stays to himself on his own farm.

I arrive at the farm later that morning. It is another beautiful sunny and warm day in May. I drive up his driveway and stop at the house. It is a massive and sturdy farmhouse. It has withstood many years of occupancy but is in obvious need of repairs.

I walk to the side door of the house and knock loudly. Even-

153

tually, John comes to the door in his stocking feet and worn-out clothing with a tired and worried facial expression. He tells me that the cow he would like me to see is out on the back pasture where his herd is grazing. He insists that I drive him out to the pasture to find the cow. He is not able to walk that far.

John opens the passenger door of my car and makes himself comfortable in the passenger seat. He directs me to drive out his back lane to the pasture. As we stop in front of the entrance gate, he exits the car and struggles to open the worn wooden gate. I drive through and wait patiently for him to close the gate and reenter my car. Every movement he makes is slow and painful. I can see that this experience is going to take a lot of time.

We start driving through the pasture. The pasture is grown up with tall grasses, weeds, low-growing shrubs, and even a few small trees. It has not been mowed for several years, not by intention, but by neglect.

We search through the grass and underbrush for the cattle. I drive carefully as I do not know what obstacles are hidden in the brush for the detriment of my vehicle.

Occasionally we find a cow/calf pair hidden in the underbrush. As we pass each cow paired with her calf, he tells me all he can remember about each of them. He knows every animal. They are his family. Every cow has a story. He remembers them well. Some have been with him a long time and have long histories. Others are younger with shorter stories. He has named them all. He tells me who their mother is and her name.

He knows their temperament. Some are tranquil and easygoing. Some are more mobile and suspicious of infringements on their space. Some can be quite aggressive. Beef cattle moms can be very protective of their calves and will defend their space aggressively. Caution is appropriate when approaching a mom with her calf by her side. He tells me when they were born. He knows their health history.

These are Herford cows. Their faces are covered with white hair. Their bodies are covered with patches of red and white hair. The pattern of those patches is unique to each cow or calf. Those patterns allow John to uniquely identify each cow as an individual.

As he identifies and tells a story about each cow, a calmness overcomes him. I see that these cattle are his friends. He loves them. His demeanor relaxes as we encounter them in the jungle of his pasture. He is in no hurry. He is enjoying the experience of viewing his family.

I remember that his call this morning is to examine a sick cow. We have not found her yet. Time is passing quickly as we meander around his back pasture. I ask him if he knows where the sick cow is at this time. John responds that he is not sure but he still has a feeling that one of them is sick. We need to continue our search for her.

I plow ahead with the cautious backcountry tour of his pasture and I play along with small talk as he narrates each cow with her story. Eventually, we have covered every square foot of his pasture. I have not seen any cows that appear sick. They all seem to be content as they graze on the green spring grass and nurse their calves on this warm, beautiful day in the month of May.

I ask John if we have accomplished the mission. Does he still think there is a sick cow among the herd? He agrees that they all look healthy and well. He seems more relaxed and the worried expression has left his face. He seems re-energized as a smile creeps across his face.

We drive back to the house. He thanks me graciously as he exits the car with a broad and gentle smile as he walks back to his house. I drive out his driveway knowing that the real purpose of this farm call was to drive him through his pasture to see his friends. He needed to see them to be content they were well.

Weeks later, I see John's obituary in the newspaper. It is a brief listing of the usual relatives and a short mention of his farming career. There is no reference to his life accomplishments or involvements in the community.

We all have a life story. They contain episodes of accomplishments, failures, successes, regrets, laughter, sadness, lifelong relationships, broken relationships, hopes, and unfulfilled dreams. They are set in a lifeline story as the years pass.

The story is built with every opportunity or barrier that comes before us. Some people have more opportunities than others. Some have mostly barriers. It would be great if life was fair. However, it is not. It never has been fair. Part of the story is our response to what we encounter. We can respond with gratitude or resentment, thankfulness or bitterness, anger or joy. The choice of how we respond is ours. These emotions are part of our spirit.

People throughout the ages have searched for a spiritual purpose to their existence. Those that believe in a spiritual reality find purpose in discovering God. They find Him as a friend that knows their story. They find Him as a loving parent that watches over a child.

As time passes, the story is interrupted with God encounters. The more they search for Him the more they see Him. When they fail to search, they do not find Him. They see the times He has protected them. They see the times they have wandered away and He has waited patiently for them to turn back to Him. God knows our story. He wants to be part of it. He wants the whole story to be occupied by Him. However, He has granted us free will to choose our own path. We determine the details and outcome of our story.

As one reads through the story of the Israelites in the Old Testament, we can see a storyline that is occupied by similar struggles that people have always faced. Their history is full of the types of struggles of spirit that we still face today. There are times of obedience and blessing. There are times of disobedience and wandering from God with resulting hardship and abandonment. However, one theme remains. God never leaves them. He brings circumstances, sometimes severe hardship, to draw them back into His fold. He wants them back. Actions have consequences. We benefit or suffer based upon our choices. It is all part of their story. It is all part of our story.

Epilogue

You have made it this far to the end of this book. The stories I tell are all inspired by my real-life experiences. I am humbled by the life God has given me. I often wonder how I got to where I am at. It has not been so much by my own self-inspired effort as it has been by the opportunities that God has placed before me. I only need to recognize these as opportunities and not as obstacles. Many times the things that are the most frustrating when they occur are the same things that are a true blessing in their outcome.

Life is a timeline of gaining more or losing more. It depends on our awareness and attitude towards the daily challenges. I can fret about something I do not like, or I can search for the opportunity within that challenge. The glass can be half empty or half full.

Viktor Frankl was in the Auschwitz Concentration Camp in 1943. As he said, "No one can take from me the freedom to choose how I will respond to what happens to me."

God has granted everyone the same freedom to make choices. He has given us a hunger in our souls. It is a hunger to know a spiritual reality. We are given a choice to decide how we respond to that hunger. We can deny it by ignoring it and going on our own path. We can rationalize that the hunger is just an age-old story not relevant today. We can replace it with the distractions of acquiring wealth and the pursuit of personal pleasure. We can bury that hunger by the pride we take in what we see as our own accomplishments. Yet, the hunger remains.

Ultimately, the only food that will satisfy that hunger with an undeniable peace within our soul is to come to grips with knowing God and the life He offers us. We do that by accepting the gift He gave us through Jesus. The evidence that the spiritual hunger has been satisfied is a peace within us. It is a confidence that there is a spiritual reality beyond this physical life. It is a confidence in knowing that we will graduate to a place that is eternal because it is timeless. The spiritual reality that God offers us is a place that is not bound by the dimensions of length, depth, height, and time. It is the final chapter in our life story.

I am reminded of experiences I had during a trip to Central Asia serving as a guest advisor to dairy farms in Kazakhstan. The people were very nice. They loved to entertain with their customs. We would all recline seated on the floor around a huge Persian rug for a celebratory meal. It is the custom for the hosts to receive a toast from the guest before the meal. The guest is given the cooked head of a goat. The guest is to bite off the ear of the goat and offer a toast of blessing to the hosts.

The toast of blessing I offer the reader is to become a seeker to satisfy the hunger of their soul. Seek an absolute truth that is not contaminated by the agendas of surrounding culture. It does not come by way of mass media outlets, social platforms, or pressure from peers. It can only come from a seeking within their soul, an awareness of the truth God reveals within us to those who earnestly seek Him. When one persists in seeking and discerning God, He will meet them with His spirit.

The irony of this book is that it appeals to the rational to discover that which appears to be beyond earthly reason. God gives humans a desire and a mind capable of finding Him. He gave us minds of reason. With effort, we can use that reason to discover that it is more reasonable to believe in God than to not believe in Him. That starts a lifelong adventure of discovering God's revelation to each individual person that dares to reach beyond the boundaries of humanly-acquired knowledge for that greener grass of spiritual wisdom.